Social Representations, Health and Illness

"This book provides a very instructive overview of the origins, development and fruitfulness of social representations theory and research. With its international and well-structured focus on research in various domains of health and illness, this is a perfect source for illustrating the usefulness of the approach for doing studies in these fields. As it also presents in detail the various methodological approaches used with this approach in these fields, it is a very valuable resource not only for researchers but also for teaching in social and health psychology and the health sciences beyond."

—Uwe Flick *Professor, Qualitative Social and Educational Research, Freie Universität Berlin, Germany*

"This is an authentic work, fully in line with the theoretical and methodological paradigm of social representations. Drawing on a large number of empirical studies in several countries and cultural contexts in Europe and around the world, with young and older adults, the author takes an exemplary grasp of his subject—health and illness. A book fully in line with the effort to understand from the inside a system of social representations that guide everyday behaviour, influenced by contact with others, communication, and culture, in the effort to experience one's body, age, health and illness in the real world. A fascinating read for experts, students, but also curious laypeople."

—Nikos Kalampalikis *Professor of Social Psychology, Lyon 2 University, France*

Michael Murray

Social Representations, Health and Illness

History, Development and Change

palgrave
macmillan

Michael Murray
School of Psychology
Keele University
Staffordshire, UK

ISBN 978-3-031-98493-8 ISBN 978-3-031-98494-5 (eBook)
https://doi.org/10.1007/978-3-031-98494-5

This Palgrave Macmillan imprint is published by the registered company Springer Nature Switzerland AG.
The registered company address is: Gewerbestrasse 11, 6330 Cham, Switzerland

"This book is a major contribution to the area of how art, culture, humanity and intellectualism, in the context of social and political conditions, helps in the further development of research and clinical work in social and health psychology."

—*Ad A. Kaptein,* Emeritus Professor of Medical Psychology, Leiden University, The Netherlands

Acknowledgements This book appears after much prevarication. Over the years, I have discussed the ideas with many people, some of whom are now sadly deceased. I would like to acknowledge, in chronological order, the many individuals who have influenced my research trajectory. First and foremost was Ivana Marková, who encouraged me to critically engage with social psychological theory and continued to inspire me throughout my career. She introduced me to Rob Farr, who alerted me to the work of Claudine Herzlich and Serge Moscovici. Then I met Beulah Bewley, who turned my interest to public health issues. Uwe Flick and Kerry Chamberlain have both continued to enthuse me about qualitative methods, while David Marks has reminded me of the importance of social context. I would like to thank Neil Tilley, who encouraged me to explore participatory action research; Cathy Campbell for her work on community health psychology; Mike White and Mark Webster for promoting my interest in community arts; and Ad Kaptein for reminding me of the importance of arts in general. A particular thank you to Ari Väänänen, who has inspired me to adopt a historical and cultural perspective. I would also like to thank Roger Beech, Mim Bernard, Paul McGarry, Judith Sixsmith and Ryan Woolrych for promoting my interest in research with older people. This multi-disciplinary heritage is reflected in the text.

At the core of this book are a series of research projects that I had the good fortune to work on over many years. I would like to thank all of the people who agreed to participate in the various projects. Their contributions to the many individual interviews, discussions, and surveys have been invaluable and form the basis of much of the work discussed.

In particular, I would like to thank Mark Johnson, Linda Jarrett, and Tony Swan, with whom I worked on the smoking study, which was funded by the Medical Research Council; Carol McMillan, who worked with me on the study funded by the Ulster Cancer Foundation; Daryl Pullman, Theresa Heath, and Monique Goguen-Campbell, who worked with me on the Norms and Narratives study funded by the Social Sciences and Humanities Research Council of Canada; Neil Tilley, Barbara Neis, and Stephen Bornstein, with whom I worked on several studies funded by the Canadian Institutes for Health Research; and Sian Maslin-Prothero, Tom Scharf, Amanda Crummett, David Amigoni, Lucy Munro, Jill Rezzano, Friederike Ziegler, Liz Postlethwaite, and Alex Lamont, with whom I had the opportunity of working on different projects funded by the New Dynamics of Ageing Research Programme. Many, many other people were involved at various stages of these projects, including assisting with obtaining finance, organizing access to resources, assisting with the collection and analysis of the qualitative and quantitative data, and many other tasks. I would like to thank them all. Many thanks also to my former students, including Billie-Jean Flynn, Anne Kearney, Kelly Monaghan, Katie Wright-Bevans and Jennifer Taylor, for persevering with my rambling thoughts.

In preparing this manuscript, I was grateful for the many comments I received from my good friends Ad Kaptein and Ari Väänänen. A particular thank-you goes to the detailed commentary provided by one of the anonymous reviewers and to Grace Jackson, Beth Farrow and Clelia Petracca of Palgrave Macmillan for their belief that I would actually finish this manuscript, and to Connie Li and Christy Michael for ensuring I got over the final hurdles. Last, but not least, I would like to thank Matthew and Daniel for their encouragement, and Anne for her unswerving support, in sickness and in health, over many years.

Contents

List of Figures

List of Tables

CHAPTER 1

Introduction

Health is an intrinsic part of being human. The United Nations' 1948 Universal Declaration of Human Rights states: 'Everyone has the right to a standard of living adequate for the health and wellbeing of himself and of his family' (United Nations, 1948). But what do we mean by health? This is a challenge that philosophers and scientists have pursued for centuries.

The World Health Organization struggled with this quandary and concluded with a much-quoted definition as 'a state of complete physical, mental and social wellbeing and not merely the absence of disease and infirmity' (Schamme, 2023). This grandiose definition was drafted in 1948 and reflected the idealism of the times just after the Second World War, when society was striving to begin to build a new peaceful world. Robert Gauthier, who was Secretary-General of the League of Nations Health Organization and was involved in developing the definition, linked the ideas of health and social change in an accompanying document, stressing that 'now is the time for aiming at positive health and social justice' (in Larsen, 2022).

Since then, there have been many developments in society and in health care. While this is an ideal definition of health, what does it mean in everyday life? This is the challenge posed by this book. Its central theme is exploring the contribution of social representation theory to deepening our understanding of health and illness. Social representation theory is concerned with exploring the social dynamics of shared

M. Murray, *Social Representations, Health and Illness*,
https://doi.org/10.1007/978-3-031-98494-5_1

understandings of the world. This approach has a certain history, and to appreciate its contemporary relevance requires an understanding of the historical context. Although it is an approach that was developed by Serge Moscovici in France in the 1950s, it can be traced back to earlier quests to investigate shared understandings of reality. In many ways, this historical perspective is comparable to the nineteenth-century German psychologist Hermann Ebbinghaus, who described psychology as having a long past but a short history (Farr, 1996). While many researchers have focused on the short history of psychology, often tracing it to Wilhelm Wundt's laboratory in Leipzig in 1879, there were many earlier attempts to understand human thought and actions. Similarly, while many researchers into social representation theory trace its development to post-war France, there were many earlier attempts to explore shared understandings of reality.

This book develops a social psychological approach to understanding lay representations of health and illness, which is distinct from the cognitive information-processing approach developed by Howard Leventhal and his colleagues (Leventhal et al., 1980; Petrie & Weinman, 1997). That so-called self-regulation approach to understanding illness has gained wide currency within health psychology. Its popularity has been accelerated by the development of a number of measures of illness perceptions that are based upon this approach (e.g., Moss-Morris et al., 2003; Weinman et al., 1996). That approach has largely ignored the social context and conceptualized these lay representations as purely cognitive constructs (Murray, 1990, 1993; Ogden, 1995). Recognizing this deficiency, its originators (Leventhal et al., 1997) have remarked: 'The self-regulation framework needs to be extended into the social context. Doing so will allow us to return to Thomas and Znaniecki's (Thomas & Znaniecki, 1918) original conceptualization of attitudes as shared beliefs' (p. 39). This book provides an opportunity to extend the idea of attitudes as shared beliefs.

The study of social representations of health and illness also has a history, from the original work of Claudine Herzlich in France through the plethora of studies that have been published subsequently. Finally, my own research on social representations of health and illness has a history, from research into smoking among young people in the Midlands of England in the 1970s and early 1980s, through the study of health and cancer in Ireland in the late eighties, to the study of ageing among baby boomers in Canada in the early 2000s, and the study of older people in the

English Midlands in the 2010s, along with many other studies in between. Since social representations are immersed in their socio-cultural context, an understanding of this corpus of research requires an exploration of the changing context.

This book is organized into three sections. The first part consists of an exploration of social representation theory and associated research methods. There are many other books that have explored this theory in detail (e.g., Flick, 1998; Jovchelovitch, 2007; Marková, 2023; Moscovici, 2000) but this book attempts to position it within its social and historical context. In that sense, it explores the background of social representation theory, its key proponents and their personal histories, and how they have further developed the theory and its methods of research. In doing so, the aim is to emphasize that this is not a theory that emerged out of thin air but has a certain heritage. It further explores the cultural and intellectual context within which the original ideas and subsequent research developed.

The theory developed in the 1950s, but it had sustained historical forebears, and it is for this reason that I have spent some time tracing its origins and the context within which it emerged. Over the years, the details of this theory have evolved, and the methods it has preferred have developed. This part of the book is intended as a guide to the next two parts, which consider empirical work.

The second part introduces research on social representations of health and illness from childhood through to old age. It is not intended to be a comprehensive review of the relevant literature, as there has been an explosion of research in this area. Rather, this section introduces some key research and also details some of my own research in this area. Some of this research has been published within an explicit social representation framework. Other research has remained confined to a series of largely descriptive reports, which have been mined and re-interpreted to reveal the importance of social representation theory. The sequence of chapters in this section moves from the study of social representations of health and illness in childhood, through to its study among adults, and then to its study among older people. Each of the studies considered is placed within its socio-cultural context, with reference to the heritage of the lead researchers. This emphasizes that our understanding of health and illness changes as we develop and in different historical periods.

The central study detailed in Chap. 4 was part of a much larger project that explored smoking among adolescents and young people, conducted in the English Midlands in the 1970s and 1980s. Much of the original project employed survey methodology and has been reported in a series of journal articles. The later part of this study adopted interviews and considered not only smoking but also young adults' views on health and illness. Some of this work was published in a monograph (Murray and McMillan, 1988) but this publication is now out of print. I have looked back on this work as well as additional details from the interviews.

The central study reported in Chaps. 5 and 6 was part of a project focused on cancer screening that was conducted in Northern Ireland during the 1980s. That study involved interviews and focus groups with a sample of men and women, coupled with a large questionnaire survey. Some of the questionnaire findings have been published (Murray & McMillan, 1993) but the findings from the interviews and focus groups have been consigned to a series of reports. Chapter 5 presents some of the findings from the reports on women's views of health and illness (Murray, 1988) while Chap. 6 considers their views on cancer (Murray & McMillan, 1987).

Chapter 6 reports some of the findings from the Norms and Narratives Study of changing views on health, illness and ageing that was conducted in Canada in the early 2000s (Murray et al., 1999). This study involved a series of focus groups, followed up by individual interviews with a large sample of baby-boomers. Some of the initial findings from this study have been published (Murray et al., 2003) but others have remained in a series of reports. Several of these reports (Murray & Rodgers, 2002) are considered in this chapter. All of the original findings have been reviewed from the perspective of social representation theory.

The final section begins with a consideration of how researchers can start to explore changes in social representations of health and illness. Again, I focus on some of the research in which I have been involved, especially that which has examined the value of arts-based methods. Some of the research discussed has been described in several journal articles (Bernard et al., 2015; Murray & Crummett, 2010; Murray & Tilley, 2006) but much of it has remained in research reports (Murray & Dolomount, 1994; Murray & Rodgers, 2005).

In her book *In Memory of Memory,* Maria Stepanova described some of the challenges of writing about past events. She sifted through photographs, memoirs and many other sources in an attempt to make some sense of her past. It was not enough to record these or place them in a sequence. The challenge was to interpret them and to provide some sort of narrative coherence to the many events. This is where we search for an interpretive framework: 'When the foundations of our day-to-day life subside and shift, hindering any attempt at systematic interpretation, we begin to search out handrails, and to welcome even the merest hint of structure'. We bring to old research some new ideas but also carry with us the shadow of old ideas. As Stepanova reflected: 'Any story about myself became a story about my ancestors. There they were behind me like an opera chorus encouraging my aria—only the music was written seventy years ago' (Stepanova, 2017, p. 99).

The underlying theme of the book is that to explore social representations of health and illness, we require an understanding of the socio-cultural (historical and developmental) context within which the social representations develop. This is not to say that social representations are epiphenomena, but rather that their character is immersed in, yet also contributes to, that context. Social representations are dynamic social constructions. They draw upon current and past experiences and shape our understanding of our everyday world.

The book is the result of an attempt to bring the findings from several projects together. This was not my initial intention when I started on the research trail, but rather, looking backwards, I have attempted to look for connections and to develop some sort of narrative coherence. So, the book as a whole is also, in part, a story of my research trajectory over the past forty or so years. An Eastern wise man once remarked that old researchers often have few new ideas but simply repeat old ideas in different ways throughout their life history. Perhaps, in considering these ideas in different settings, their value can become clearer.

References

Bernard, M., Rickett, M., Amigoni, D., Munro, L., Murray, M., & Rezzano, J. (2015). Ages and stages: The place of theatre in the lives of older people. *Ageing & Society, 35*, 1119–1145.

Farr, R. M. (1996). *The roots of modern social psychology*. Oxford: Blackwell.

Flick, U. (Ed.). (1998). *The psychology of the social*. Cambridge University Press.

Jovchelovitch, S. (2007). *Knowledge in context: Representations, community and culture*. Routledge.

Larsen, L. T. (2022). Not merely the absence of disease: A genealogy of the WHO's positive health definition. *History of the Human Sciences, 35*(1), 111–131.

Leventhal, H., Benyamini, Y., Brownlee, S., Diefenbach, M., Leventhal, E. A., Patrick-Miller, L., & Robitaille, C. (1997). Illness representations: Theoretical foundations. In K. J. Petrie & J. A. Weinman (Eds.), *Perceptions of health and illness* (pp. 19–45). Harwood Academic.

Leventhal, H., Meyer, D., & Nerenz, D. (1980). The commonsense representations of illness changes. In S. Rachman (Ed.), *Contributions to medical psychology* (Vol. 2). Pergamon.

Marková, I. (2023). *The making of a dialogical theory: Social representations and communication*. Cambridge University Press.

Moscovici, S. (2000). *Social representations: Explorations in social psychology* (G. Duveen, Ed.). Polity.

Moss-Morris, R., Weinman, J., Petrie, K., Horne, R., Cameron, L., & Buick, D. (2003). The revised Illness Perception Questionnaire (IPQ-R). *Psychology and Health*, *17*(1), 1–16.

Murray, M. (1990). Lay representations of illness. In P. Bennett, J. Weinman, & P. Spurgeon (Eds.), *Current topics in health psychology* (pp. 63–92). Harwood Academic.

Murray, M. (1993). Social and cognitive representations of health and illness. In H. Schroder, K. Reschke, M. Johnson, & S. Maes (Eds.), *Health psychology—potential in diversity* (pp. 124–131). S. Roderer Verlag.

Murray, M. & McMillan, C. (1993). Gender differences in perceptions of cancer. *Journal of Cancer Education*, 8(1), 53–62.

Murray, M., & Crummett, A. (2010). 'I don't think they knew we could do these sorts of things': Social representations of community and participation in community arts by older people. *Journal of Health Psychology*, *15*, 777–785.

Murray, M., & Dolomount, M. (1994). *A constant danger: Accidents among fishermen*. Division of Community Health, Memorial University.

Murray, M., & McMillan, C. (1987). *Working class women's views of cancer*. Prepared for Ulster Cancer Foundation.

Murray, M., & McMillan, C. (1988). *Working class women's views of health, illness and the health service*. Prepared for Ulster Cancer Foundation.

Murray, M., Pullman, D., & Rodgers, T. H. (2003). Social representations of health and illness among baby-boomers in Eastern Canada. *Journal of Health Psychology*, *8*(5), 485–499.

Murray, M., Pullman, D., Turner, L., & Simpson, E. (1999). *Norms and narratives: Beliefs regarding health in an ageing population, research proposal*. Social Science and Humanities Research Council.

Murray, M., & Rodgers, T. H. (2002). *Atlantic Canada baby-boomers' representations of health, illness and aging: Norms and narratives, research report II*. Memorial University, NL, Canada.

Murray, M., & Rodgers, T. H. (2005). *"The fishing will never ever leave me": Injured fish harvesters talk about accidents, injuries and disability*. SafetyNet, Memorial University.

Murray, M., & Tilley, N. (2006). Using community arts to promote awareness of safety in fishing communities: An action research study. *Safety Science, 44*, 797–808.

Ogden, J. (1995). Changing the subject of health psychology. *Psychology and Health, 10*, 257–265.

Petrie, K. J., & Weinman, J. A. (Eds.). (1997). *Perceptions of Health and Illness*. Harwood Academic.

Schramme, T. (2023). Health as complete well-being: The WHO definition and beyond. *Public Health Ethics, 16*(3), 210–218.

Stepanova, M. (2017). *In memory of memory*. Fitzcarraldo.

Thomas, W. I., & Znaniecki, F. (1918). *The Polish peasant in Europe and America*. Badger.

United Nations. (1948). *Universal declaration of human rights*. Retrieved March 19, 2025, from https://www.un.org/en/about-us/universal-declaration-of-human-rights.

Weinman, J., Petrie, K. J., Moss-Morris, R., & Horne, R. (1996). The illness perception questionnaire: A new method for assessing the cognitive representation of illness. *Psychology and Health, 11*, 431–446.

PART I

History, Theory and Methods

CHAPTER 2

Origins of Social Representation Theory

Since ancient times, scholars have attempted to conceptualize how we make sense of our world. Social representation theory is a contemporary approach concerned with the understanding of the world shared by a community or society. This approach was initially developed in the 1950s by the French social psychologist Serge Moscovici. Since then, many researchers have sought to develop it theoretically and to consider its applications. This chapter considers its historical forebears and contemporary developments. It also identifies some of the key figures in the development of the theory, whose work will be considered in subsequent chapters.

2.1 Backstory

Ideas develop and change during different historical periods. The study of how humans make sense of their worlds has been a central concern for generations of philosophers and psychologists. Different researchers have developed various approaches. These ideas are connected to distinct historical periods. This book focuses on some specific European developments.

In the fifth century BCE, at the time of the Greco-Persian wars, the Greek philosopher and historian Herodotus, who could also be described as an early social psychologist, discussed a distinction between the thinking

M. Murray, *Social Representations, Health and Illness*,
https://doi.org/10.1007/978-3-031-98494-5_2

of 'Greeks' and 'non-Greeks'. In his *Histories*, written about 450 BCE, he wrote about the purpose of his work as being 'to prevent the traces of human events being erased by time and to preserve the fame of the important and remarkable achievements of both Greeks and non-Greeks; and more particularly, the cause of hostilities between the Greeks and non-Greeks'. This focus on the achievements and thinking of different peoples arose out of concern about the conflict between them and has been a recurring issue for researchers for centuries. Herodotus placed great emphasis on the importance of *nomos*, which can be translated as custom or culture. He gave as an example the ancient Athenian custom of cremating their dead relatives in contrast to certain Indian communities who preferred cannibalism. The Greeks and Indians respected the method preferred within their own community, while they reacted with revulsion to the preference of the other community. This illustrated not only the importance of custom but also the role of shared beliefs within different cultures (Humphreys, 1987).

With the development of European nation-states in the seventeenth and eighteenth centuries, philosophers extended their discussion of what differentiates one group from another and how this changes over time. The Italian philosopher Giambattista Vico (1668–1744) wrote about the common sense shared by a society at a certain period, which is reflected in its literature, language and philosophy. He also discussed changes in ways of thinking throughout history and how people of his era were able to engage in scientific thinking, unlike the Ancients. Changes in the character of ideas were linked with changes in the structure of a society, and he noted how ideas evolve over time. However, this was not a one-way process. Rather, as Vico stated in the aptly titled *New Science*: 'But in the night of thick darkness enveloping the earliest antiquity, so remote from ourselves, there shines the eternal and never failing light of a truth beyond all question: that the world of civil society has certainly been made by man' (see Simon, 1981, p. 318). We are not pawns in history; rather, we create our own history, to an extent. Marková (2016) summarized Vico's thinking: 'Human beings create their common senses by humanising nature in and through actions, by establishing communities, social institutions, traditions and political organisations'. She continued: "Underlying agreements" that underlie common sense have therefore meanings only if they are considered in the historical analysis of ideas in which humans have created themselves (p. 49).

Moving into the nineteenth century, the study of national differences became more extensive in Europe. There developed broad political debate on the so-called German question, which was concerned with the best political way to integrate the 37 then-independent German-speaking states in central Europe. Of particular note was the work of the German philosopher Moritz Lazarus (1824–1903), who, in 1851, introduced the term *Völkerpsychologie* to characterize the shared understandings of ordinary people, which he argued typified the emergent German nation. Lazarus's term was an attempt to identify what exactly unified the German people beyond language. The very term is difficult to translate and is concerned with the everyday psychology of ordinary people.

In 1859, Lazarus, together with the linguist Heymann Steinthal (1823–1899), established the *Zeitschrift für Völkerpsychologie und Sprachwissenschaft* [*Journal of Völkerpsychologie and Linguistics*], which brought together an interest in the shared knowledge of peoples with the study of languages. A more social and communicative approach to exploring national differences began to develop. The aim of this new approach was to unite the natural sciences with the humanities to develop an understanding of the historical development of the folk spirit (*der Völksgeist*) that typified the nation, as expressed through its language, myths, religion, customs and habits. As Lazarus and Steinthal argued in 1855: 'Man is by birth a member of a *Völk*, and is thus determined in his mental development in manifold ways. The individual cannot be completely comprehended without regard to the mental whole (*die geistige Gesamtheit*) in which it has been created and in which it lives' (Klautke, 2013, p. 18). For them, a nation was a social phenomenon that developed around this collective spirit (*Gesamtheit*), and it was through this process that its residents developed a collective sense of identity. Although language was central to this process, a nation could share several languages. To accommodate this diversity, Lazarus and Steinthal argued that an important factor was the subjective view of the people—that they shared the same identity and the same customs and habits. It was through this emphasis on the subjective criterion and shared customs that they strove to integrate Jewish and other minority ethnic groups within the broader German identity.[1] The importance of elucidating the strength of national identity and of nationalism continues today (e.g., Storm, 2025).

[1] On the front of the German parliament building in Berlin is the phrase *Dem Deutschen Volke* (The German People).

Lazarus and Steinthal emphasized that they drew upon the ideas of the great German philosopher Georg Hegel (1770–1831). In particular, they drew upon his concept *objektiver Geist* (objective spirit or objective cultural mentality), which Hegel developed as part of his study of personhood. *Geist* refers to the shared mentality of mankind, or what Solomon (1970) termed a 'general consciousness' (p. 642). The German philosopher Heymann Steinthal (1823–1899) noted that 'Whoever does not recognise the concept of *objektiver Geist* in *Völkerpsychologie* understands nothing of its history' (in Brock, 1992, p. 209). Hegel's notion of a shared mentality approach was opposed to that of individualism. He also argued that the way we think is ultimately shaped by our history. We cannot escape from our time and place. He viewed his own philosophy as a child of its time (Hutchings, 2015).

Wilhelm Wundt (1832–1920), who has often been considered the father of experimental psychology, took up the idea of shared mentality at the University of Leipzig in Germany. Besides his experimental work, he was interested in exploring broader social phenomena using non-experimental methods. The focus of his research was on the ethnographic study of everyday life, language, culture, myths and religion, which he detailed in his multi-volume *Völkerpsychologie*. Central to this psychology were three pairs of basic concepts: *Volkgeist* and *Volksseele* (collective spirit and collective mind), *Vorgeschichte* and *Geschichte* (prehistory and history), and *Einzelne* and *Gemeinschaft* (individual and community). He emphasised the individual and shared ways of thinking, which were socially and historically located. For Wundt, 'the core characteristic of the collective mind [. . .] lies in the continuity of psychological processes that go beyond an individual's life span' (Wong, 2009, pp. 246–247). Here, he was stressing the importance of historical processes.

In 1927, Eleanor Wundt compiled a catalogue of Wundt's extensive writings. In reviewing this, Wong (2009) noted that Wundt had 'grounded *Völkerpsychologie* on the dialectical relationship between individual (*Einzelne*) and community (*Gemeinschaft*)' (p. 248). The way to investigate these processes was through two approaches. The first was the comparative-psychological approach, which studied historical and ethnological phenomena from a psychological perspective. The second was the historical-psychological approach, which considers the historical context of psychological processes. Unfortunately, these approaches were ignored in the rush to develop a scientific psychology, which was guided by measurement and experimentation. Today, the development of multiple qualitative approaches within psychological research has begun to redress this orientation.

The concept of *Völkerpsychologie* has sometimes been condemned as racist, and Wundt has even been decried as a racist. However, Wundt had no interest in studies of national character (Brock, 1992). Rather, he was interested in exploring shared psychological processes that were immersed in history and society. Furthermore, his confreres, Lazarus and Steinthal, were not only Jewish but also active in the struggle against anti-Semitism and were hostile to attempts to define *Völk* in biological terms. It was a social and cultural phenomenon.

The nineteenth century was a period of sustained social upheaval throughout Europe. Karl Marx (1818–1883) was interested in the movement of the proletariat into political action. He did not explicitly refer to Wundt's work but was interested in how ideas differed between social groups. He described how certain social groups or classes maintained their power in society not just by material force but by the power of ideas. It was for this reason that he and Friedrich Engels (1820–1895) argued in *The German Ideology* ([1846] 1968):

> The ideas of the ruling class are in every epoch the ruling ideas, i.e. the class which is the ruling material force of society, is at the same time its ruling intellectual force. The class which has the means of material production at its disposal, has control at the same time over the means of mental production, so that thereby, generally speaking, the ideas of those who lack the means of mental production are subject to it. The ruling ideas are nothing more than the ideal expression of the dominant material relationships, the dominant material relationships grasped as ideas (p. 21).

Marx and Engels claimed that, to grasp how people make sense of the world, we need to consider both the material basis and the power relationships between social classes. While Marx drew upon Hegel in the development of his approach, he strongly criticized Hegel for what he considered his idealist approach. He claimed he had inverted Hegel's ideas by basing them in material reality. Marx, however, stressed the importance of Hegel in developing the idea of dialectics, as he said in *Capital.*

> The mystification which the dialectic suffers in Hegel's hands by no means prevents him from being the first to present its general forms of motion in

> a comprehensive and conscious manner. With him, it is standing on its head. It must be inverted, in order to discover the rational kernel within the mystical shell (Marx, [1867] 1963, pp. 102–103).

Although Marx did not refer to Wundt, he did briefly mention Vico (in a footnote, Marx, [1867] 1963). Both thinkers were concerned with history and the role of conflict. Marx thought such conflict could be positive, whereas for Vico it held out the possibility of chaos. Further, while Vico emphasized the role of non-material and linguistic-communicative factors in making history, Marx stressed the importance of material factors (Ball, 1994). However, as Moscovici later emphasised Marx did not claim that material factors were sufficient (see below).

Later Marxists were aware of the work of Wundt. Vladimir Lenin (1870–1924) referred to him frequently in his discussion of 'materalism and empirio-criticism' (Lenin, 1909). He accepted that Wundt had written extensively on everyday thinking but concluded that he 'adheres to an idealist viewpoint' (p. 61). Although he sympathetically described Wundt as 'that old bird', he dismissed him as being full of the 'ballast of professorial erudition, with superfluous niceties and reservations' (p. 62). In his defence of dialectical materialism, Lenin explicitly attacked Wundt's ideas as idealist and detached from material reality but remained convinced that his study of collective processes was important (Brock, 1992).

Many psychologists and social scientists came to Leipzig to study with Wundt. Among these was Émile Durkheim (1858–1916), who was particularly interested in Wundt's concept of *Völksseel*, or the shared understanding of reality. Durkheim (1898) distinguished between individual and collective representations of the world. The former, he argued, was the concern of psychologists and focused on cognitive processing, whereas the latter was the province of sociologists and was concerned with beliefs and ideas that are developed and shared by a collective but are not reducible to individual constituents. Such collective representations distinguished one collective, such as a nation, from another. Individual representations were 'variable, fleeting, and short-lived', whereas collective representations were 'impersonal and untouched by time' (Rateau et al., 2012, p. 481). These ideas had a broad resonance within the developing social science community.

The nineteenth century also saw the growth of contact between European and other civilizations, particularly in Africa and South America, and with it, the growth of social science disciplines such as anthropology, devoted to understanding these new peoples. The French anthropologist

Lucien Lévy-Bruhl (1857–1939) took up Durkheim's ideas of collective representations to explain how the way of thinking of 'primitive' peoples differed from that of modern peoples. For example, Lévy-Bruhl (1922) argued that 'primitive' people have collective representations about the causes of disease, which they attribute to supernatural forces and believe to be self-evident and part of their symbolic worlds (Klautke, 2013). Their thinking was rational when considered within these symbolic worlds.

Meanwhile, in North America, there was a rapid growth of immigration from Europe by people often fleeing starvation and poverty. The sociologist William Thomas (1863–1947) opined that 'further advances in certain lines of individual psychology and social philosophy were dependent on "reliable generalisations" from folk psychology' (Thomas, 1896, in Klautke, 2013, p. 37). Later, he produced, with Florian Znaniecki (1882–1958), the multi-volume *The Polish Peasant in Europe and America* (1918). The Polish immigrants to America were often impoverished peasants and were known as *za chlebem* ('for bread') immigrants. Thomas and Znaniecki's research was concerned with studying the attitudes of these peasants toward their dramatically changing world. These two researchers conceptualized attitudes not as an individual phenomenon but as a social phenomenon, as something that was shared by a collective (see Farr, 1996; Murray, 2002).

An important figure in the development of social psychology in North America was George Herbert Mead (1863–1931), who had also spent time in Leipzig with Wundt. He eagerly read Wundt's *Völkerpsycholgie* and used some of the ideas in the development of his social psychology. He was particularly interested in the role of language and social interaction as the basis of human consciousness (Farr, 1983).

Back in Europe, the Austro-Hungarian Empire was a fertile ground for the development of new ideas. One of these was psychoanalysis and the search for the hidden roots of human behaviour. Both Sigmund Freud (1856–1939) and Carl Gustav Jung (1875–1961) were interested in Wundt's anthropological work, especially his work on the shared thinking of people. Freud (1919) described Wundt's work as the stimulus for his discussion of the *totem* as the emblem of a group. He was also interested in how psychoanalytic concepts could be applied to exploring shared folk psychology and traditions. Of particular importance was Freud's exploration of the unconscious, that part of the mind which he claimed was not accessible through introspection but could influence our everyday life (Power, 2000).

Jung, who was influenced by the work of Lévy-Bruhl, extended these ideas to explore the collective unconscious, which he distinguished from Freud's personal or individual unconscious (Segal, 2007). This collective unconscious consisted of 'primordial images' or 'archetypes,' which are shared by humanity. Jung suggested that it consisted of the psychic life of our ancestors, stretching back in time. This was comparable to Wundt's concern with historical processes.

In the twentieth century, Jean Piaget (1896–1980), who had studied under Jung while in Zurich, explored the development of understandings of the world among children. He termed this process 'lay epistemology,' which he investigated in his study of the thinking of his own children. Piaget was aware of the work of both Lévy-Bruhl and Durkheim. Later, Moscovici (1998a) traced this connection: 'Without exaggerating one can say that psychology of "primitive" representations established by the French thinker [Lévy-Bruhl] is repeated in the psychology of children's representations (for example, in childhood animism, intellectual realism, etc.) which we owe to the Swiss psychologist [Piaget]' (p. 227). Piaget was also knowledgeable about Marx, and they were both convinced of the importance of human agency in explaining consciousness. As Wartofsky (1982) noted:

> Both Piaget and Marx begin with the premise that the forms of human consciousness are shaped by praxis, by the modes of human action; that the conscious subject is not the passive recipient of external impressions; that ideas are not simply copies of reality; that human beings are agents active in the transformation of the world in accordance with their needs and interests, and thereby agents in their own self-transformation (p. 470).

Although Piaget did consider the role of social interaction in cognitive development, there was less attention to the role of the social and cultural context. At one stage, he wrote, 'there are neither individuals as such nor society as such. There are just inter-individual relations' (Piaget, 1977, in Muller & Carpendale, 2000). Moscovici was later keen to explore lay epistemology, but within its social and cultural context.

A contemporaneous group of philosophers who were interested in how we make sense of the world were the phenomenologists. A key figure was the Austrian philosopher Edmund Husserl (1859–1938), who attended classes by the phenomenologist Franz Brentano (1838–1917) and was concerned with how we see the world itself rather than the world as an object to be studied (Langdridge, 2007). An important aspect was that we are always intentionally aware of something in the world. Phenomenological psychology is concerned with detailing this awareness of something. Husserl was interested in Lévy-Bruhl's work on collective representations. Serge Moscovici later referred to a letter that Husserl had written to Lévy-Bruhl in 1935:

> Of course, we have long known that each human being has their 'representation of the world', that each nation, each supra-national cultural sphere lives so to speak in another world than that which surrounds them, and we also know that is the same for each historical period (Moscovici, 1998a, p. 223).

He was again emphasizing the importance of the historical context of ideas.

Martin Heidegger (1889–1976) extended Husserl's approach but argued that it was not possible to focus on the true essence of experience and bracket off other influences. Instead, we must be aware of the historical and cultural context within which the perceiving occurs. Marková (2024) noted that Heidegger also distinguished between thinking as a dynamic process and non-thinking as fixed states of mind. According to her, Heidegger emphasized that 'although all people have the capacity to think, they are often thoughtless. It is thinking that defines humanity and therefore, the more thoughtless we are the less human we are' (p. 796). This distinction between the content and dynamic nature of thinking is something to which we will return. However, Heidegger's Nazi connections should not be ignored and confirm what Moscovici later noted that the most rational minds can still be infected by murderous ideas (see below).

Fritz Heider (1896–1988), the Austrian-American who developed attribution theory in the 1950s, drew upon the Austrian/German phenomenological tradition. He noted that a key influence in his education was Alexius Meinong (1853–1920), who took the idea of intentionality from Brentano. According to this conception, all mental concepts are directed at something. Heider commented: 'I have always had the conviction that thought and perceptions are "about" something in a way that the fall of a stone is not "about" anything' (Heider, 1983, p. 21). He went on to develop his 'naïve psychology', 'which gives us the principles we use to build up our picture of the social environment and which guides our reactions to it' (Heider, 1958, p. 5). This resulted in his classic work *The Psychology of Interpersonal Relations* (Heider, 1958) in which he argued that 'the ordinary person has a great and profound understanding of himself and of other people which, though unformulated or only vaguely conceived, enables him to interact with others in more or less adaptive ways' (p. 2). It was this concern with the everyday thinking of ordinary people that was at the centre of social representation theory. However, unlike Moscovici, who emphasized the importance of everyday social interaction, Heider declared that his work 'will center on the *person* as the basic unit to be investigated' (p. 1).

In France, these ideas on perception were further developed by Jean-Paul Sartre (1905–1980) and Maurice Merleau-Ponty (1908–1961), who promoted an existential phenomenology that is concerned with the meaning of human existence. These ideas came to prominence shortly after the end of the Second World War and reflect the turmoil of the French people contemplating their experiences of resistance and collaboration. Sartre argued that we are constantly involved in creating our lived existence. His ideas are summarized in his classic lecture *Existentialism and Humanism,* which was published in French in 1946 and in English two years later. His primary idea was that 'man (sic) is condemned to be free' (Sartre, [1948] 1970, p. 34). More specifically, 'Condemned, because he did not create himself, yet is nevertheless at liberty, and from the moment that he is thrown into this world he is responsible for everything that he does' (p. 34). But we are also social beings, such that 'it is not only one's own self that one discovers in *cogito*, but those of others too' (p. 45). Further, we have a moral responsibility for others. As he says: 'freedom as the definition of a man does not depend upon others, but as soon as there is a commitment, I am obliged to will the liberty of others at the same time as mine' (p. 52). Moscovici (2019) recalled that in his early years in Paris: 'Existentialism remained the dominant French philosophy as if anxiety was the ethos of the time'[2] (p. 102, trans.). An indication of the popularity of these ideas in French society was that when Sartre died in 1980, about 50,000 mourners walked in his funeral cortege.

Merleau-Ponty, who was both a philosopher and a psychologist, emphasized the central role of the body in perceiving the world. This forms the basis of later discussions about embodiment and the concern with how consciousness is embedded in the body. Merleau-Ponty was also concerned with meaning-making, or making sense of the world. The

[2] 'L'existentialisme restait alors le fleuron de la philosophe française, comme si l'angoise résumait l'ethos de l'époque'.

person is a *corps-sujet*, a lived body. He argued that we are 'condemned to meaning' because of our very location in the world (Langdridge, 2007). He criticized Piaget's view of children's cognitive development as proceeding from illogicality to logicality and argued that children's thinking was adapted to their lived experience (see Marková, 2024, p. 797). This connecting of the psychological with the social would later become central to social representation theory. His ideas on embodiment are still being developed and have potential applications for understanding social representations of health (Weiss & Haber, 1999).

These philosophical and psychological ideas preceded the development of social representation theory by Serge Moscovici in the 1950s. He developed his theory from these earlier ideas but emphasized the dynamic character of socially shared knowledge—not as something that was the fixed property of the individual or the collective, but rather as the result of the active engagement of people in everyday social interaction that was socially and historically located. It was a social psychological phenomenon. To understand Moscovici's interest in these ideas, it is important to consider the historical context. As he himself (Moscovici, 1998b) said later: 'We can have as many Piagets and Vygotskys as we want if our understanding of their work is not anchored in its historical context' (p. 413). He further added the need to explore not only the social and political context but also the broader intellectual context. There is 'a common tendency to search for the source of a theory within psychology itself. As if, in our science, one did not borrow or find inspiration in ideas and principles from other sciences' (p. 413). For Moscovici, a crucial issue was the nature of modernity—the character of modern society (Taylor, 1991).

2.2 Beginnings of the Theory

Serge Moscovici was born in Romania into a Jewish merchant family in 1925. His father separated from his mother when he was young, and he lived much of his subsequent early years with his father until he reached adolescence. Eastern Europe, including Romania, had witnessed sustained persecution of Jewish people in the nineteenth century. With the rise of fascism across Europe in the 1930s, there were renewed attacks on Jewish communities. In Romania, there were ongoing clashes between the anti-Semitic Iron Guard and other political groups. When he was only 13 years of age, Moscovici was expelled from his high school following the introduction of anti-Semitic legislation in the country. Instead, he attended a vocational school studying mechanics.

During the Second World War, the Romanian government sided with Hitler, and attacks on the Jewish population increased dramatically. According to the Wiesel Commission (2004), between 280,000 and 380,000 Romanian and Ukrainian Jewish people in Romania were murdered or perished in various circumstances during the war. A further 135,000 Romanian Jews living in Northern Transylvania also perished. The Commission concluded:

> Of all the allies of Nazi Germany, Romania bears responsibility for the deaths of more Jews than any country other than Germany itself. The murders committed in Iasi, Odessa, Bogdanovka, Domanovka, and Peciora, for example, were among the most hideous murders committed against Jews anywhere during the Holocaust. Romania committed genocide against the Jews. The survival of Jews in some parts of the country does not alter this reality.

Many Jewish people, including Moscovici, avoided death but were interned in forced labour camps.

It was this experience of persecution and tyranny that encouraged him and many others from his background to join the then-illegal Communist Party at the age of 16. He was following the resistant path of his uncle, Ilie Moscovici, who was a leader of the Romanian Social Democratic Party. Moscovici later traced his theoretical ideas to his early experiences of oppression and injustice and his efforts to challenge it. He was fascinated by how ideas could spread rapidly throughout a society and how a minority could have a disproportionate influence.

He eagerly read not only political thought but also philosophical and literary works. In his memoir *Chronique des années égarées* (Moscovici, 1997) he recalled the early impact of the thinking of the French philosopher Blaise Pascal (1623–1662), who, in his *Pensées*, placed belief and thought at the centre of his philosophy. Pascal compared human life to a 'thinking reed'. He argued that 'It is not in space that I should search for my dignity, but in the control of my thoughts ... The universe comprehends me by space and engulfs me like a point; by means of thought, I comprehend it' (Clarke, 2015). His most famous argument, described as 'Pascal's wager', placed belief at the centre of human understanding. He argued that belief in

God is more advantageous than non-belief, since, if it is true, one can subsequently reap the reward. Much later, Moscovici asserted that 'the biggest mystery in life is the power of beliefs [. . .] It is through belief that every indifferent thing and every neutral thing can be transformed into a passion' (Moscovici & Marková, 1998, p. 397). Here, he was reflecting on how one can become passionately committed to certain activities through the power of belief in certain ideas. From this, he became interested in how formalized bodies of knowledge can be grasped and transformed into everyday beliefs and the prospect of collective action:

> It is when knowledge and technique are changed into beliefs that they bring people together and become a force which can transform individuals from passive members into active members who participate in collective actions and in everything which brings existence in common alive (Moscovici, 1998a, p. 214).

In 1944, Moscovici was freed from forced labour by the advancing Red Army and became involved in various activities, helping refugees make their way out of Romania to various countries, including the nascent state of Israel in Mandatory Palestine. At that time, it was estimated that there were over ten million refugees from all nations moving around Europe. In this post-war period, European society was in a state of flux, and new identities were being formed. In 1947, at the age of 22 and frustrated by the continuing anti-Semitism he experienced under the new Communist regime in Romania, Moscovici decided to leave his home country and made his way across Europe to Paris, which was regarded as the intellectual centre of Europe at that time.

When he came to Paris in 1947, he initially worked in various manual jobs and, at the same time, read widely, discussing various ideas with the many intellectuals who were attracted to that city. He described this phase of his life vividly in an autobiography that was constructed after his death from notes he had kept (Moscovici, 2019). The clash of scientific and political ideas that he encountered fascinated him. The role of science was of widespread interest among his colleagues. Later, he noted that 'we were all interested to know in what way science had an impact on our technical thinking and on our material prospect' (Moscovici & Marková, 1998, p. 374). This interest in science was particularly pronounced among those who had a more critical orientation: 'all young people who were attracted by Marxism, communism and socialism were aware that those were the dominating issues' (p. 374). Moscovici was interested in how these ideas were transformed into everyday thinking. As he said: 'My experience during the war made me wonder about the impact of science on ordinary culture, how it changes the minds and behaviour of people, how it becomes part of our belief systems, and so on' (Moscovici & Marková, 1998, p. 375).

The role of science in society intrigued him. In a subsequent interview, he noted: 'The problem for me was the following: How is scientific knowledge transformed into common, ordinary, or spontaneous knowledge?' (Moscovici & Marková, 1998, p. 375). But what is science? Moscovici considered it an abstract body of knowledge, but it did not occur out of thin air. As he explained:

> Anyone who is familiar with the history of the sciences knows that most highly abstract theories and notions first occurred to scientists or science in a figurative mode, and that they were laden with symbolic, religious, political or sexual values (Moscovici, 2008, p. 21).

In his autobiography, Moscovici recalled how he grappled with conceptualizing this process of making sense of science. There was little discussion of the concept of common sense in the social science literature at that time, but then he came across a work on the French polymath Marin Mersenne (1588–1648) by the cleric Robert Lenoble (1902–1959), which had been published in 1946. In his work, Lenoble wrote: 'There is no common sense but as many common senses as civilization'[3] (Ohayon, 2015, trans.). Different societies have different common senses. Moscovici was intrigued by this formulation and subsequently recalled it as the impetus for his later work: 'but in an instance, I recognised the concept that I was looking for'[4] (Moscovici, 2019, p. 202, trans.).

While Moscovici was concerned with how common sense engaged with scientific ideas, he was also aware that scientific ideas were not fixed, and that there was an intermingling of different ideas. Later, he referred to Durkheim's interest in the role of religion (see Moscovici, 1998a, p. 215):

> law, morals, and scientific thought itself were born in religion, were long confounded with it, and have remained imbued with its spirit (Durkheim, [1921] 1995, p. 65).

[3] 'Il n y a pas de sens commun mais autant de sens communs que le civilization'.

[4] 'mais en un instant, j'a vais reconnu le concept que je chercerais'.

Although he had lost his own religious faith, he was still intrigued by how it mixed with the thinking of ordinary people and its power over their lives.

In Paris, after the war, many psychologists were influenced by Marxist ideas and concerned with broad social issues. The Communist Party, which had played an active role in the Resistance movement, was very strong, and Moscovici initially thought about studying the extent to which Marxism had been transformed into everyday thinking. However, he decided that it was not a good idea 'to start a social scientific research with a politically charged issue' (Moscovici & Marková, 1998, p. 377), especially as he was a new arrival in France. He decided instead to focus on psychoanalysis, which at that time was extremely popular in French society and could be considered a mixture of science and religion. Besides, his supervisor, Daniel Lagache (1903–1972), who had introduced him to social psychology, was a psychoanalyst. Lagache also introduced him to the ideas of various contemporary social thinkers. The classmates of Lagache at the École Normale had included both Sartre and Merleau-Ponty (Herzlich, 2018).[5] Moscovici later recalled that while he was interested in phenomenological ideas, he found them too static and wanted to develop an approach that was more socially dynamic (Moscovici & Marková, 1998, p. 393). He later described these early days of his research as his 'age of innocence', since at that time there was little social psychology in Europe and he did not have any contact with researchers in the field. However, this period of intellectual freedom allowed him to read widely across the social sciences and humanities.

He was particularly incensed by the idea that only scientists and intellectuals could think rationally and wanted to understand how ordinary people grasped and transformed scientific ideas. Moscovici said that this interest had grown during his wartime experiences. It was through his contact with the communist movement and his critique of the basic Marxist approach to the way of thinking of ordinary people that his ideas developed. He argued that, from a Leninist perspective, ordinary people's thoughts were filled with folk irrationalities and had to be replaced with scientific knowledge. Their irrational thinking could be transformed

[5] In 1955, Lagache established a new sub-discipline which he termed 'psychology in health settings', which preceded by many years the later formal development of health psychology in the English-speaking world. His approach was inspired by psychoanalytic ideas (Santiago-Delefosse & del Rio Carral, 2018).

through propaganda. Moscovici contrasted this approach with what he considered the Enlightenment perspective. According to this perspective, scientific knowledge could dispel folk irrationalities by means of communication and education. Moscovici felt that both the Marxist and the non-Marxist perspectives considered the thinking of the ordinary person as being irrational, which could be transformed either by propaganda or education.

This was the root of Moscovici's quest to develop an alternative perspective: 'I reacted against the underlying idea which had preoccupied me for a long time: namely against the idea that people do not think rationally' (Moscovici & Marková, 1998, p. 375). He continued: 'In fact, one could say that it is the intellectuals who do not think rationally, having produced such irrational theories as racism and Nazism' (p. 375). Indeed, he recalled that he had written about this problem in 'an adolescent essay [...] immediately after the war. In that essay, I criticized the Marxist duality or opposition concerning science and ideology as the roots of social consciousness. I supported the view that there is a third component or factor there: common sense' (p. 375–376).

After the horrors of the Second World War, Moscovici was keen to explore why so many people had succumbed to fascist ideas. Like many others, he thought that perhaps psychology would provide some answers. After completing a basic licence in psychology in 1949, followed by a diploma at the Institute of Psychology at the Sorbonne, he began work on his doctorate in 1951. His research focused on how scientific and professional knowledge, in his case psychoanalysis, was transformed into everyday knowledge. Through this research into the nature of common sense, he developed his theory of social representations that was both theoretical and applied.

He did this both through talking with ordinary people and also through analysing popular newspapers of both the Catholic Church and the Communist Party. It would be 10 years before Moscovici finally presented his thesis for defence (Ohayon, 2013). The 1950s was a period of sustained post-war reconstruction in France, and it was in these difficult times that Moscovici strove to conduct his research. He defended his thesis in 1961 and published it as a book the same year (Moscovici, 1961). Fifteen years later, another version was published (Moscovici, 1976, 2008).

An important early influence on Moscovici was the work of Marx and various Marxist thinkers. At the beginning of the 1961 edition, he quoted the Russian Marxist Georgi Plekhanov (1856–1918), stating that 'there is no historical fact that does not have its origin in the economy of society; but it is no less true that there is no historical fact that is not preceded, accompanied and followed by a certain state of consciousness. Hence the importance of social psychology'[6] (Moscovici, 1961, p. 4, trans.). Plekhanov (1976) maintained a continuing interest in the role of social psychology in understanding ideas in their historical context.

Moscovici (1961) cautioned that Marx had not definitively posited that material factors were of prime importance. He argued that 'Marx and Engels never announced this theory, but only put forward a hypothesis on the socio-economic conditioning of intellectual productions, leaving concrete research—which they only began—to clarify the consequences that result from it'[7] (p. 339, trans.). However, he was hostile to what he considered to be Lenin's dismissive view of the 'common thinking' of ordinary people. For Moscovici, the primary quest was the understanding of everyday thinking and communication.

After the Russian Revolution, many Soviet psychologists, such as Lev Vygotsky (1896–1934) and Alexander Luria (1902–1977), began to explore the social and historical roots of everyday thinking. Moscovici (1998a) noted how they were aware of the work of Lévy-Bruhl. He quoted from Luria (1976, p. 7):

> Lévy-Bruhl was the first to point out the qualitative feature of primitive thought and the first to treat logical processes as products of historical development. He had a great influence on psychologists in the 1920s who tried to go beyond simplistic notions about the mind and to understand human consciousness as a product of sociocultural development.

It was for this reason that Luria and his colleagues conducted research among the supposedly primitive peoples of Central Asia to explore the socio-cultural context of everyday thinking.

[6] 'pas un fait historique que n'ait son origine dans l'économie de la société; mais il est non moins vrai qu'il n'est pas un fait historique qui ne soit précédé, accompagné et suivi d'un certain état de la conscience. D'où l'importance énorme de la psychologie sociale' (Moscovici, 1961, p. 4).

[7] 'Marx et Engels n'ont jamais énoncé cette théorie, mais seulement avancé une hypothèse sur les conditionnements socio-économiques des productions intellectuelles, laissant aux recherches concrètes—qu'il ont seulement entamées—le soin d'éclaircir les consequences qui en découlent' (Moscovici, 1961, p. 339).

From Lévy-Bruhl, the French social anthropologist, Moscovici drew upon the ideas of the rationality of everyday thinking. Lévy-Bruhl was keen to clarify the rationality of so-called 'primitive' cultures. Later, Moscovici (1998b) summarized Lévy-Bruhl's thinking: 'Social representations are rational in the eyes of members of one culture, they need not be so, either in the same sense or according to the same logic, in the eyes of another culture [...] it is impossible to convert superior forms of thought, chosen by one culture, into universal laws of the human mind' (p. 417). He argued that Lévy-Bruhl's ideas were the catalyst for the initial work of Jean Piaget and Lev Vygotsky.

Moscovici also drew upon the phenomenological ideas of Merleau-Ponty and the work of Fritz Heider. Much later, he recalled: 'When I wonder today about what has crystallized this notion of representation in my mind, I think I was reading Merleau-Ponty' (Moscovici, 1990b, p. 233). He had attended some classes by Merleau-Ponty and drew upon his ideas about perception but aimed to transform it into a social process. He was also aware of the work of Heider, who at that time was developing his ideas on naive psychology, which guides everyday social interaction. Later, Moscovici (1998a) noted that Heider's focus on perception ignored the 'beliefs, language or the meanings embedded in this language' and characterized it as 'acultural and ahistorical' (p. 239), neglecting the importance of context.

Jean Piaget was very important in his thinking, as he was concerned with how children make sense of the world. Moscovici recalled that he drew upon Piaget's theoretical as well as methodological ideas. Besides the influence of Merleau-Ponty, he also claimed that it was Piaget who introduced him to the concept of representation: 'In reading Piaget, it occurred to me that I could try to study common knowledge in adults just as Piaget studied it in children, but I took the view that this common knowledge resulted from transformation of another kind of knowledge' (Moscovici, 1998a).

A particular innovation that Piaget introduced was that children begin to grasp the world through the processes of assimilation and accommodation. The former is concerned with the integration of new information into established cognitive frameworks, while the latter is concerned with how new information can change and develop new frameworks. Moscovici developed the concepts of anchoring and objectification as two central processes in the development of social representations. While anchoring is the process by which new information is transformed by connecting it to more familiar concepts, objectification is the process by which abstract concepts are given meaning by transforming them into something more concrete. These processes are central to explaining the development of social representations, as we will discuss later.

Although the 1961 publication attracted considerable attention in France, Moscovici's interests shifted in the following decade when he pursued work on social influence. This was concerned with the study of those activities which lead to social change. He was particularly interested in the influence of the minority. He returned to developing his ideas on social representation theory in the 1970s. In the intervening period, he was very active in organizing the European Association of Experimental Social Psychology (EAESP), which was formally established in 1966 with Moscovici as Chair, followed by Henri Tajfel (1919–1982) in 1969 (Moscovici & Markovà, 2006).

After the devastation of the Second World War, the 1950s, when Moscovici conducted his research, marked the beginning of tremendous economic growth in France. It was known as the *Trente Glorieuses*[8]—the Thirty Glorious Years. The Communist Party had initially entered into government with De Gaulle and helped to establish the Fourth Republic. However, in the 1950s, they were excluded from government and adopted a more resistant stance with respect to American influence. Psychoanalysis was perceived as a malign force in French society. Moscovici explored this representation in the Communist press and contrasted it with that in the Catholic press. The Catholic Church was also hostile to psychoanalysis but found ways of reconciling some aspects with its beliefs. In addition, Catholics could see some similarities between their religion and the practice of psychoanalysis, such as parallels between therapy and confession.

There were tensions between psychoanalysis and the Communist and Catholic belief systems. As Moscovici argued: 'When an idea or scientific knowledge enters into the field of culture, of society, then you can have real cultural fights, intellectual fights' (Moscovici & Markovà, 1998, p. 377). It was this process of conflict between belief systems that particularly interested Moscovici (1998a, p. 394). Compared with attitudes, social representations are a much broader phenomenon. Indeed, 'the representation is what holds attitudinal items together' (Moscovici &

[8] *Les Trentes Glorieuses* was the title of an influential book by Jean Fourastié (1979), which detailed the rapid changes in French society post-war.

Marková, 1998, p. 381). Social representations can contain conflicting attitudes and ideas. Those which come to prominence will depend upon the social circumstances.

It was in this climate of intellectual tension in the 1950s that Moscovici described his quest as not 'in developing a social psychology of cognition in the sense of social perception or social memory, etc. What I wanted to develop was *a social psychology of knowledge*' (Moscovici & Marková, 1998, p. 381). He wanted to understand both the structure and processes underlying common sense, sometimes described as lay epistemology or the 'thinking society' (Flick, 1998a).

He published the second edition of his thesis in 1976. In the preface, he continued his criticism of the dominant approach in social psychology, which restricted its concern to the study of individuals and small groups. He added that another inadequacy was the 'positivist philosophy, for which the only things that matter are forecasts that can be empirically verified and phenomena that can be observed directly' (Moscovici, [1976] 2008, p. xxiii). The study of social representations would expand beyond these restrictions in epistemology, theory, and method.

Moscovici placed the study of social representations within its social and historical context. In the Foreword to the original edition, Lagache also commented on how the social representation of psychoanalysis described by Moscovici was a child of its time and would have been different from that apparent if the study had been conducted in the 1920s (Lagache, 1961, p. xxi). In his Preliminary Remarks to the 1976 edition, Moscovici noted that 'increasingly, it is through the intermediary of other people that we are familiarized with theories and phenomena, and we cannot verify them on the basis of individual experience' (Moscovici, [1976] 2008, p. xxvii). In the Afterword to that edition, he remarked on the continuing societal changes and noted a growing individualism in French society and the greater attention being paid to private life and intersubjective relations (p. 363). Similarly, the Canadian philosopher Charles Taylor, in his discussion of modernity, has commented on the increasing individualism in the late twentieth century:

> the dark side of individualism is a centering on the self, which both flattens and narrows our lives, makes them poorer in meaning, and less concerned with others or society (p. 4).

In this second 1976 edition, Moscovici ([1976] 2008) identified Durkheim as being of prime importance in the development of his ideas. Durkheim had distinguished between individual and collective representations to describe how ideas circulated in society. The former was the property of individual cognition and of interest to psychologists, while collective representations were those collective belief systems that typified different societies. These collective representations are backed by authority and are the dominant ideas in a society. Conversely, Moscovici argued that social representations were the result of the active engagement of people in everyday social interaction. They change over time, but they also impose themselves on communities and distinguish one community from another.

The 1961 edition emphasized the importance of language and communication in the construction of social representations. That edition relied less on Durkheim and more on a range of social and psychological thinkers. This difference between the two editions of the original thesis has led to some confusion. The second edition is more widely available and has been translated into English, while the first French edition is more difficult to access, leading to a greater emphasis on the ideas of Durkheim, which are highlighted in the second edition.

In the first edition, Moscovici (1961) stressed the importance of Marxist ideas, especially of ideology, in the development of interest in the sociology of knowledge (p. 5). As previously mentioned, he referred to the Russian Marxist philosopher Georgi Plekhanov, who had written extensively on the role of social psychology in explaining social change. There is limited reference to Plekhanov in the second edition, although there remained extensive reference to Marx. Moscovici ([1976] 2008) highlighted the importance of history in his Afterword to the second edition, where he quoted Marx's famous remark from *The Eighteenth Brumaire of Napoleon Bonaparte*: 'Men make their own history, but they do not make it just as they please; they do not make it under circumstances chosen by themselves, but under circumstances directly encountered, given and transmitted from the past' (Marx, [1852] 1968, p. 97; Moscovici, [1976] 2008, p. 362). An understanding of history was important in understanding how people make sense of their worlds. Fifteen years after the publication of the first edition, Moscovici was here stressing the importance of the historical context of his original work.

2.3 Early Developments

Moscovici developed the basic ideas of social representations theory in the 1950s, and they were quickly expanded upon by some of his co-workers in France. From an early stage, Moscovici involved various researchers in his work. These individuals subsequently developed their own research trajectories, and their work continues to influence the development of social representations theory.

One of his earliest colleagues was Claudine Herzlich, who worked on Moscovici's classic study of psychoanalysis in the 1950s. Herzlich went on to develop her own study of social representations of health and illness, which we will consider in subsequent chapters. Of particular note was the foreword that Moscovici (1973) wrote in the monograph that resulted from her thesis (Herzlich, 1973). In it, he summarized the basics of social representation theory. He began by emphasizing the socially dynamic nature of social representations:

> First of all, there is no implication of any clear-cut division between the outside world and the inner world of the individual (or group); subject and object are not regarded as functionally separate. An object is located in a context of activity, since it is what it is because it is in part regarded by the person or the group as an extension of their behaviour (p. xi).

He then proceeded to provide a more detailed description of the phenomenon:

> A social representation is a system of values, ideas and practices with a twofold function; first, to establish an order which will enable individuals to orientate themselves in their material and social world and to master it; and secondly to enable communication to take place among members of a community by providing them with a code for social exchange and a code for naming and classifying unambiguously the various aspects of their world and their individual and group history (p. xiii).

This much-quoted definition clearly defines not only the content of social representations (viz., a system of values, ideas and practices) but also its function (viz., enabling individuals to orientate themselves and to communicate with others). It is also noticeable that, in his reference to 'practices' as being part of social representations, he expanded the concept beyond the symbolic level.

Another researcher at *École pratique des hautes études (EPHE)* was Denise Jodelet. She co-authored a textbook on social psychology in 1970, which included a preface by Moscovici on psychosociology. In the first edition of his foundational work, Moscovici (1961) had noted: 'Our description of the social representation frankly accentuated its psychosociological character'[9] (p. 311, trans.). This reference to psychosociology indicated his expansive approach to social psychology.

In 1976, Jodelet published, with Moscovici, a report entitled *La Représentations Sociale du Corps,* confirming Moscovici's interest in representations of the body (Herzlich, 2018). Jodelet's doctorate was delayed, but finally, in 1985, she completed her thesis on social representations and mental illness and published it as a monograph titled *Folies et Représentations Sociales* in 1989. An English version of this research, titled *Madness and Social Representations. Living with the Mad in One French Community,* was then published two years later (Jodelet, 1991) and will be discussed in subsequent chapters. Here, it is important to highlight her contribution to exploring not simply the ideas and values within social representations but also the practices. Jodelet continued to develop a more sociocultural approach to the study of social representations (Madiot et al., 2008).

An important influence on both Jodelet and Herzlich (2018) was the anthropologist Claude Lévi-Strauss (1908–2009), who had returned shortly after the war to Paris after gaining a position at *EPHE,* where they worked. In 1962, he published his classic work *La Pensée Sauvage* (*The Savage Mind*, Levi-Strauss, 1966) in which he detailed his ideas on human thought: 'In this book it is neither the mind of savages nor that of primitive or archaic humanity, but rather mind in its untamed state as distinct from mind cultivated or domesticated for the purpose of yielding a return' (Levi-Strauss, 1966, p. 219). This anthropological heritage accords with Herzlich's (1973) description of her work as 'partly anthropological and partly psychosociological in its approach' (p. 3). Additionally, Moscovici (1961) remarked on the relationship between anthropology and social psychology and noted that 'research in the human sciences that falls within a strictly defined context is rare'[10]

[9] 'Notre description de la représentation sociale accentue franchement son caractère psychosociologique'.

[10] 'les recherches dans les sciences humaines qui s'incrivent dans un context strictement défine étant rares'.

(p. 14, trans). Much later, he described his view of social psychology as 'an anthropology of the modern world' (Moscovici, 1990b, p. 169).

Another early researcher in Moscovici's laboratory was Willem Doise (1935–2023), who completed his doctorate in 1967. After he moved to Geneva, Doise subsequently went on to develop his influential levels of explanation approach in social psychology, in which he distinguished between intra-personal, interpersonal, positional and ideological explanations (Doise, 1986) and the organizing principles approach to social representations (Doise et al., 1993), which we will consider later.

2.4 Spreading Interest

Over the following years, Moscovici attracted dozens of young researchers to Paris, where he had established the *Laboratoire Européen de Psychologie Sociale* within the EPHE. Many of these researchers have had an enduring impact on expanding the remit of social representations theory. Research centres with a focus on social representations theory developed throughout Europe, especially in France, Italy and Portugal.

In Latin America, interest in social representation theory grew substantially, particularly in Brazil, but also in Argentina, Mexico and other countries. Jodelet played a key role in promoting this interest. In her review of presentations at the international conferences on social representations, which have been held every two years since 1992, Annamaria de Rosa (2019) found that Brazil had the most active research activity, even more than France. Reflecting the importance of community and liberation psychology in Latin America, concern with social representations there has taken up issues of social conflict, power and social change (de Sousa & Oswald, 2021).

Within the English-speaking world, by the 1960s, there was growing reflection within social psychology and the social sciences regarding both epistemological and methodological issues (Armistead, 1974; Murray, 2014, 2018). In 1963, Peter Berger and Thomas Luckmann had published *The Social Construction of Reality,* which provoked discussion about the social nature of reality (Berger & Luckmann, 1963). In 1973, Ken Gergen published his influential paper on 'Social Psychology as History', in which he argued that theories of social behaviour are reflections of historical processes (Gergen, 1973).

Moscovici contributed to this debate. The book *The Context of Social Psychology* (Israel & Tajfel, 1972) included a chapter by Moscovici (1972) on a plan to invigorate the study of social psychology. This volume also included chapters by Tajfel (1972) on the social context of experiments and another by the Czech psychologist Jaromír Janoušek (1972) on the concept of praxis in Marxist thought. Together, these chapters illustrate the desire to expand the remit of social psychology both methodologically and theoretically into a discipline that was more social and political.

Moscovici's (1972) chapter criticized the disinterested stance of much of social psychology, with its concern for scientific respectability and ignorance of societal issues. Instead, he asked the questions: 'What is the aim of the scientific community? Is it to support or to criticize the social order? Is it to consolidate it or to transform it?' This is almost a repetition of Marx's famous Eleventh Thesis in his critique of the German philosopher Ludwig Feuerbach: 'Philosophers have hitherto only *interpreted* the world in various ways; the point is to *change* it' (Marx, [1845] 1924). Marková (2023) noted the influence of Marx and argued that Moscovici 'viewed social psychology as a political science both in terms of its theories and practice and as a discipline in movement that should play a significant role in society' (p. 19). He later produced a volume on social influence for the book series (Moscovici, 1976) illustrating his desire to promote a more socially engaged psychology.

Although Moscovici (1972) did not explicitly refer to social representations in this chapter, he briefly referred to his thesis, 'which described the extent to which psychoanalytic theory has penetrated common sense in everyday judgements, discussions and interpretations of people's actions' (pp. 37–38). He also placed the study of common sense at the centre of a revitalized social psychology:

> The proper domain of our discipline is the study of cultural processes which are responsible for the organization of knowledge in a society, for the establishment of inter-individual relationships in the context of social and physical environment, for the formation of social movements (groups, parties, institutions) through which men act and interact, for the codification of inter-individual and intergroup conduct which creates a common social reality with its norms and values, the origin of which is to be sought again in the social context (p. 55).

It is this concern with understanding common social reality that formed the focus of social representation theory. However, the concern is not simply to describe the content of social representations but also their internal dynamics. Later, Moscovici (1984) summarized this endeavour:

> Social psychology, on the other hand, is and must be preoccupied solely with both the structure and the dynamics of representations. For us, it is summed up in the difficulty of penetrating the interior to discover the inner mechanisms and vitality of social representations in the greatest possible detail: that is in 'splitting representations', just as atoms and genes have been split" (pp. 16–17).

Of central concern was the process of the social construction of reality. This was not simply something contemporary but also drew upon history.

Despite the growing interest in social representation theory, Moscovici's classic work (second edition) had to wait until 2008 for an English translation (Moscovici, [1976] 2008). The second edition had already been translated into Portuguese in 1978, reflecting the growing interest in social representation theory in Latin America, and an Italian edition was published in 2011 (de Rosa, 2011). The delay in the publication of this key work into English may have been at least partly due to Moscovici himself. In an interview, he even claimed that, because of his cultural background, he was against proselytism. He remarked that 'there is a quasi-religious respect for knowledge in that [Jewish] culture, and if one thinks that the idea is right, one believes that it will make its way through despite the outside resistance' (Marková and Moscovici, 1978: 373–374). The delay in the eventual English translation of *Psychoanalysis. Its Image and Its Public* definitely delayed the interest in social representation theory in the English-speaking psychological community. In that community, non-English ideas were often ignored. Another important factor was the declining interest in psychoanalysis and the dominance of American social psychology, with its individualistic focus, which was apparent in its preference for research on individual attitudes and beliefs and its ignorance of broader socially shared beliefs (Fowers, 2000; Greenwood, 2004). However, some of his other works were translated quickly (e.g., Moscovici, 1993).

Interest in social representation theory grew slowly in the English-speaking world. John Greenwood (2004) has detailed how social psychology in North America became detached from understanding broad social phenomena and concentrated on an individualist model of social cognition, as well as interpersonal and group phenomena. He detailed how Floyd Allport's influential *Social Psychology* textbook (1924) considered social psychology as a form of individual psychology. Wundt's work on

Völkerpsychologie was largely neglected, and instead, the focus was on his experimental work (see Wong, 2009).

Moscovici spent considerable time in New York, specifically through his appointment at the New School for Social Research in New York, where he worked closely with Leon Festinger, who had developed the theory of cognitive dissonance. A collection was published that explored connections with social cognition theory (Deaux & Philogène, 2001) but his influence in the United States was largely through his work on minority group influence (Moscovici, 1976).

Although North American ideas dominated the emerging social psychology throughout the English-speaking world, after the Second World War, alternative ideas began to be promoted in Europe. The European Association of Experimental Social Psychology, which developed during the 1970s, began to attract UK-based social psychologists. It was through these meetings that Robert Farr (1936–2013) met Moscovici and Herzlich.[11] in 1976, he spent time in Paris and returned to London enthused with the idea of developing and promoting social representation theory. His initial publication in this field explored the connections between the work of Herzlich, Heider and Harré (Farr, 1977[12]).

Farr's plan to promote social representation theory developed when he joined the London School of Economics (LSE) in 1984 to replace Hilde Himmelweit (1918–1989). Although Himmelweit had completed a more clinical PhD with Hans Eysenck at the Institute of Psychiatry in London, she was keen to reach beyond the individualistic focus of that research when she joined LSE in 1948. After her death in 1989, a collection edited with her colleague George Gaskell was published (Himmelweit & Gaskell, 1990). This collection began with a manifesto by Himmelweit for a 'societal psychology', which reached beyond the traditional focus of social psychology on individual, interpersonal and small group research. This form of psychology would emphasize 'the

[11] In the late 10970s, Farr Was involved in a European study group on 'Historical Change in Social Psychology' with Moscovici, Carl Graumann and Leon Festinger (Moscovici & Marková, 2006).

[12] Rob Farr presented an earlier version of this paper at the British Psychological Society Social Psychology conference at York in 1976. Ivana Marková had organized a symposium on attribution theory at the conference to which Rob Farr and I contributed papers. His contribution alerted me to the importance of social representation theory. My contribution was about attribution of responsibility.

all-embracing force of the social, institutional, and cultural environments, and with it the study of social phenomena in their own right as they affect, and are affected by, the members of the particular society' (Himmelweit, 1990, p. 17). Within this societal psychology, she identified social representation theory as playing a key role: 'Social representations are important because they constitute a society's symbolic or mediated reality, which, once common currency, affects not only communication but societal and personal decision making' (p. 30).

Farr's (1990) chapter in this collection traced what he described as the 'waxing and waning of interest in societal psychology' (p. 46) during the twentieth century. He referred to Moscovici's work on social representations and its distinction from Durkheim's collective representations. In his chapter, Moscovici (1990a) continued his critique of mainstream social psychology and expressed frustration at its individualistic orientation.

At the time of Farr's appointment to LSE, he and Moscovici (Farr and Moscovici, 1984) brought out a collection on social representation theory, which was the result of an international colloquium they had organized in Paris in 1979. In the introduction, they noted that the collection aimed to 'facilitate the diffusion of knowledge of this tradition of research throughout the English-speaking world' (Farr & Moscovici, 1984, p. x). This collection was, in many ways, a marker, and Farr proceeded to promote the theory in his writings (e.g., Farr, 1987a, 1987b) and, together with his graduate students, went on to further develop social representation theory.

In the 1980s, there was much discussion in British social psychology about the nature of language. This gave rise to discursive psychology (Potter & Wetherell, 1987) which grew in influence within British social psychology. It drew especially upon the British linguistic tradition, for example, the work of John Austin (1911–1960), who was interested in speech acts in everyday life, such as acts of ordering and answering. Potter and Wetherell dismissed social representations as 'mental entities ... made up of abstract and concrete elements' (p. 139). Furthermore, they argued that 'the social in social representation is merely redundant baggage, and that representations are individual phenomena' (p. 140). They ignored the broader social concerns of social representations theory and the importance given to language and communication. Moscovici was very sympathetic to discourse analysis, but he emphasized that he was opposed to the idea of 'language *über alles*' (Moscovici & Marková, 1998, p. 405).

A more critical approach to discourse analysis, drawing upon the ideas of Michel Foucault, was developed by Ian Parker in Manchester. He moved beyond concern with discourse in interpersonal interaction to consider its role in how people think and feel, as well as the material conditions in which interactions occur. Of particular importance was the role of power in Foucault's conception of discourse and how it asserts particular versions of truth. While this discussion of power relations was important, Parker (1987) continued to characterize social representations as cognitive phenomena.

After his experiences in the Second World War, Henri Tajfel (1919–1982) became interested in the social psychological processes underlying the development of prejudice. His experimental work on the minimal group paradigm focused on the minimal conditions required for groups to differentiate and discriminate against each other (Tajfel et al., 1971). However, Tajfel was keen to explore the use of this approach in the real world and, together with John Turner, developed social identity theory, which argued that people define themselves with reference to the 'ingroup' and as distinct from the 'outgroup' (Tajfel & Turner, 1986). Later work would consider how social representation theory held the potential for exploring the content of these different group identities (e.g., Duveen & Lloyd, 1987).

Another innovation in British social psychology was the ethogenic approach developed by Rom Harré (1927–2019). He combined the concern with the detailed study of social interaction promoted by microsociology (e.g., Goffman, 1959, 1963) and the Oxford School of Philosophers, who were concerned with everyday language. This approach emphasized the importance of taking into consideration people's accounts of their actions, which should be critically interpreted (Harré, 1977; Harré & Secord, 1972). It attracted some interest in the UK in the 1970s and 1980s (e.g., Marsh et al., 1978; Murray and McMillan, 1988; Totman, 1979).

A final point was the continuing interest in attribution theory in the 1980s. This theory had important connections with social representation theory, with its concern for the everyday search for explanations and the idea of the naïve scientist. Moscovici preferred the term 'amateur scientist' and insisted that attributions must be considered within the context of social representations (Moscovici & Hewstone, 1983). Miles Hewstone spent some time working with Moscovici in the 1980s and subsequently published a review of research on attribution theory, using

Doise's four-level approach to systematize the prolific research and to emphasize the importance of the societal level (Hewstone, 1989). While emphasizing the importance of social representation theory, Hewstone cautiously concluded that he had 'probably gone further than some social psychologists would wish, in exploring attributions at the societal level' (p. 235). Despite his caution, this work further extended the connections between social representation theory and other social psychological theories.

2.5 Everyday Knowledge

This chapter sketched out the historical development of social representation theory in France and elsewhere. It outlined the historical background to different approaches to the study of shared beliefs, in particular the changing social circumstances within which these ideas were developed. It then focused on Serge Moscovici's background in wartime Europe, from which grew his interest in everyday knowledge and the power of minorities. His experience of political repression drew him to radical political ideas, but he was frustrated by what he saw as the restrictive and deterministic approach of Marxism. Later, he remarked that much of Marxism dismissed the importance of everyday ideas ('the dross of representations and beliefs', Moscovici, 1993, p. 6) and focused more on the material socio-economic conditions. While these factors were important, Moscovici was interested in exploring the importance of commonplace ideas and the socio-cultural location of those ideas. Interest in his approach was initially confined to France but gradually attracted attention elsewhere in Europe and Latin America. However, it was largely ignored within the individualistic social psychology that developed in North America, although it began to have some resonance with other social psychologists in the English-speaking world. In addition, from the 1970s, other alternative approaches within social psychology began to develop. The next chapter will consider the further development of this approach, both theoretically and methodologically.

References

Allport, F. H. (1924). *Social psychology*. Houghton Mifflin.
Armistead, N. (Ed.). (1974). *Reconstructing social psychology*. Penguin.

Ball, T. (1994). *Reappraising political theory: Revisionist studies in the history of political thought*. Oxford University Press.
Berger, P., & Luckmann, T. (1963). *The social construction of reality*. Penguin.
Brock. (1992). Was Wundt a 'Nazi'?: Völkerpsychologie, racism and anti-semitism. *Theory & Psychology*, *2*(2), 205–223.
Clarke, D. (2015). Blaise Pascal. In E. N. Zalta (Ed.) *The Stanford encyclopedia of philosophy (fall 2015 edition)*. https://plato.stanford.edu/archives/fall2015/entries/pascal/.
de Rosa, A. S. (2011). Notes in the margin to a meta-theoretical analysis of the two editions of *La Psychanalyse, son image et son public*. *Papers on Social Representations*, *20*, 36(1)–36(34). 1961–1976.
de Rosa, A. S. (2019). The story continues: For a "Biography of the Theory" through the international conferences on social representations. In S. Seidmann & N. Pievi (Eds.) *Identidades y Conflictos Sociales. Aportes y desafios de la investigacion sobre representaciones sociales*. Buenos Aires, Argentina: Editorial de Belgrano.
Deaux, K., & Philogène, G. (Eds.). (2001). *Representations of the social*. Blackwell.
Doise, W. (1986). *Levels of explanation in social psychology*. Cambridge University Press.
Doise, W., Clémence, A., & Lorenzi-Cioldi, F. (1993). *The Quantitative analysis of social representations*. Harvester Wheatsheaf.
Durkheim, E. (1898). Répresentations individuelles et representations collectives. *Revue de Métaphysique Et de Morale*, *6*(3), 273–302.
Duveen, G., & Lloyd, B. (1987). The significance of social identities. *British Journal of Social Psychology*, *25*(3), 219–230.
Farr, R. M. (1977). Heider, Harré and Herzlich on health and illness: Some observations on the structure of 'representations collectives'. *European Journal of Social Psychology*, *7*(4), 491–504.
Farr, R. M. (1983). Wilhelm Wundt (1832–1920) and the origins of psychology as an experimental and social science. *British Journal of Social Psychology*, *22*, 289–301.
Farr, R. M. (1987a). Social representations—a French tradition of research. *Journal for the Theory of Social Behaviour*, *17*, 346–369.
Farr, R. M. (Ed.) (1987b). Social representations. *Journal for the Theory of Social Behaviour*, *7*(4).
Farr, R. M. (1990). The waxing and waning of interest in societal psychology: A historical perspective. In H. T. Himmelweit & G. Gaskell (Eds.), *Societal psychology* (pp. 46–65). Sage.
Farr, R. M. (1996). *The Roots of Modern Social Psychology*. Blackwell.
Farr, R. M., & Moscovici, S. (Eds.). (1984). *Social representations*. Cambridge University Press.
Flick, U. (Ed.). (1998). *The psychology of the social*. Cambridge University Press.
Fourastié, J. (1979). *Les trente glorieuses*. Fayard.

Fowers, B. J. (2000). An Aristotelian analysis of the structure of human action. In J. Martin, J. Sugarman, & K. L. Slaney (Eds.), *The Wiley handbook of theoretical and philosophical psychology* (pp. 70–84). Wiley.
Freud, S. (1919). *Totem and Taboo. resemblances between the mental lives of savages and neurotics.* Routledge.
Gergen, K. J. (1973). Social psychology as history. *Journal of Personality and Social Psychology, 26*(2), 309–320.
Goffman, E. (1959). *The presentation of self in everyday life.* Penguin.
Goffman, E. (1963). *Stigma. Notes on the management of spoiled identity.* Penguin.
Greenwood, J. D. (2004). *The disappearance of the social in American Social Psychology.* Cambridge University Press.
Harré, R. (1977). The ethogenic approach: Theory and practice. *Advances in Experimental Social Psychology, 10*, 283–314.
Harré, R., & Secord, P. F. (1972). *The explanation of social behaviour.* Blackwell.
Heider, F. (1958). *The psychology of interpersonal relations.* John Wiley.
Heider, F. (1983). *The life of a psychologist. An autobiography.* University of Kansas Press.
Herzlich, C. (1973). *Health and illness. A social psychological analysis.* London: Academic Press (Original: *Santé et Maladie: Analyse d'une Réprésentation Sociale*). Mouton. 1969.
Herzlich, C. (2018). A journey in the field of health: From social psychology to multi-disciplinarity. *Journal of Health Psychology., 23*, 386–396.
Hewstone, M. (1989). *Attribution Theory. From collective processes to collective beliefs.* Basil Blackwell.
Himmelweit, H. (1990). Societal psychology: Implications and scope. In H. T. Himmelweit & G. Gaskell (Eds.), *Societal psychology* (pp. 17–45). Sage.
Himmelweit, H. T., & Gaskell, G. (Eds.). (1990). *Societal psychology.* Sage.
Humphreys, S. (1987). Law, custom and culture in Herodotus. *Arethusa, 20*(1/2), 211–220.
Hutchings, K. (2015). Hegel, George Wilhelm Friedrich (1770–1831). In M. T. Gibbons Ed., *The encyclopedia of political thought* (pp. 1–12). Wiley.
Israel, J., & Tajfel, H. (Eds.). (1972). *The context of social psychology. A critical assessment.* Academic Press.
Janoušek, J. (1972). On the Marxian concept of Praxis. In J. Israel & H. Tajfel (Eds.), *The context of social psychology. A critical assessment* (pp. 279–294). Academic Press.
Jodelet, D. (1991). *Madness and social representations. Living with the mad in one French community.* University of California Press.
Klautke, E. (2013). *The mind of the nation. Völkerpsychologie in Germany 1851–1955.* Berghahn.

Lagache, D. (1961). Foreword. In S. Moscovici (2008), *Psychoanalysis: Its image and its public.* [English translation of *La Psychoanalyse: Son Image et Son Public,* 1976] Cambridge: Polity Press (pp. xiix–xxi).
Langdridge, D. (2007). *Phenomenological psychology: Theory, research and method.* Pearson.
Lenin, V. I. (1909). *Materialism and empirio-criticism.* Progress.
Levi-Strauss, C. (1966). *The savage mind.* University of Chicago Press.
Lévy-Bruhl, L. (1922). *La Mentalité Primitive.* Librairie Félix Alcan.
Madiot, B., Lage, E., & Arruda, A. (Eds.). (2008). *Une Approche Engagée En Psychologie Sociale: L'Oeuvre de Denise Jodelet.* Éditions Érès.
Marková, I. (2016). *The dialogical mind. Common sense and ethics.* Cambridge University Press.
Marková, I. (2023). *The making of a dialogical theory. Social representations and communication.* Cambridge University Press.
Marková, I. (2024). Book review of T. Zittoun. *The pleasure of thinking,* Cambridge: Cambridge University Press. *Culture & Psychology, 30*(3), 780–781.
Marsh, P., Rosser, E., & Harré, R. (1978). *Rules of disorder.* Routledge.
Marx, K. ([1845]1924). *Theses on Feuerbach.* Progress.
Marx, K. ([1867]1963). *Capital.* Progress Publishers.
Marx, K. ([1852]1968). *The eighteenth Brumaire of Louis Bonaparte.* Progress.
Marx, K., & Engels, F. ([1846]1968). *The German ideology.* Progress.
Moscovici, S. (1961). *La Psychanalyse: Son Image Et Son Public.* Presses Universitaires de France.
Moscovici, S. (1973). Foreword. In (C. Herzlich.), *Health and illness: A social psychological analysis* (pp. ix–xiv). Academic Press.
Moscovici, S. (1976). *Social influence and social change.* Academic Press.
Moscovici, S. (1984). The phenomenon of social representations. In R. M. Farr & S. Moscovici (Eds.), *Social representations* (pp. 3–70). Cambridge University Press.
Moscovici, S. (1990a). The generalized self and mass society. In H. T. Himmelweit & G. Gaskell (Eds.), *Societal psychology* (pp. 66–91). Sage.
Moscovici, S. (1990b). Social psychology and developmental psychology: Extending the conversation. In G. Duveen & B. Lloyd (Eds.), *Social representations and the developmental of knowledge* (pp. 164–185). Cambridge University Press.
Moscovici, S. (1993). *The invention of society.* Polity.
Moscovici, S. (1997). *Chronique Des Années Égarées: Récit Autobiographique.* Stock.
Moscovici, S. (1998a). The history and actuality of social representations. In U. Flick (Ed.), *The psychology of the social* (pp. 209–247). Cambridge University Press.
Moscovici, S. (1998b). Social consciousness and its history. *Culture & Psychology, 4*(3), 411–429.

Moscovici, S. ([1976]2008). Psychoanalysis: Its image and its public. *[English Translation of La Psychoanalyse, Son Image Et Son Image]*. Polity Press.
Moscovici, S. (2019). *Mon Après-Guerre À Paris. Chronique Des Années Retrouvées*. Grasset.
Moscovici, S. (1972). Society and theory in social psychology. In J. Israel & H. Tajfel (Eds.), *The context of social psychology. A critical assessment* (pp. 17–68). Academic Press.
Moscovici, S., & Hewstone, M. (1983). Social representations and social explanations: From the "Naïve" to the "Amateur" scientist. In M. Hewstone (Ed.), *Attribution theory: Social and functional extensions* (pp. 98–125). Basil Blackwell.
Moscovici, S., & Marková, I. (1998). Presenting social representations: A conversation. *Culture & Psychology*, *4*(3), 371–410.
Moscovici, S., & Marková, I. (2006). *The making of modern social psychology*. Polity.
Műller, U., & Carpendale, J. I. M. (2000). The role of social interaction in Piaget's theory: Language for social cooperation and social cooperation for language. *New Ideas in Psychology*, *18*, 139–156.
Murray, M. (2002). Connecting narrative and social representation theory in health research. *Social Science Information*, *41*(4), 653–673.
Murray, M. (2014). Social history of health psychology: Context and textbooks. *Health Psychology Review*, *8*, 215–237.
Murray, M. (2018). The pre-history of health psychology in the UK: From natural science and psychoanalysis to social science, social cognition and beyond. *Journal of Health Psychology.*, *23*(3), 472–491.
Murray, M., & McMillan, C. (1988). *Working class women's views of health, illness and the health service*. Prepared for Ulster Cancer Foundation.
Ohayon, A. (2013). Postface. Serge Moscovici dans l'histoire de la psychologie en France. In N. Kalampalikis (Ed.), *Serge Moscovici, Le Scandal de la Pensée Sociale* (pp. 27–290). Éditions de l'École des Hautes Études en Sciences Sociales.
Ohayon, A. (2015). À Serge Moscovici. *Nouvelle Revue de Psychosociologie*, *19*, 235–240.
Parker, I. (1987). "Social representations": Social psychology's (mis)use of sociology. *Journal for the Theory of Social Behaviour*, *17*(4), 447–469.
Plekhanov, G. (1976). *Selected Philosophical Work*. volume2.pdf (marxists.org). Vol. II Progress Publishers.
Potter, J., & Wetherell, M. (1987). *Discourse and social psychology. Beyond attitudes and behaviour*. Sage.
Power, M. (2000). Freud and the unconscious. *The Psychologist*, *13*(12), 612–614.
Rateau, P., Moliner, P., Abric, J., & Moliner, P. (2012). Social representation theory. In *Handbook of theories of social psychology* (Vol. 2, pp. 477–497). Sage.

Santiago-Delefosse, M., & del Rio Carral, M. (2018). The rapid expansion of (mainstream) health psychology in France: Historical foundations. *Journal of Health Psychology, 23*(3), 372–385.

Sartre, J.-P. (1970). *Existentialism and humanism.* Methuen. [1948].

Segal, R. A. (2007). Jung and Lévy-Bruhl. *Journal of Analytic Psychology, 52*(5), 635–658.

Simon, L. H. (1981). Vico and Marx: Perspectives on historical development. *Journal of the History of Ideas, 42*(2), 317–331.

Solomon, R. C. (1970). Hegel's concept of "Geist". *Review of Metaphysics, 23*(4), 642–661.

Storm, E. (2025). *Nationalism. A world history.* Princeton University Press.

Tajfel, H. (1972). Experiments in a vacuum. In J. Israel & H. Tajfel Eds., *The Context of Social Psychology. A Critical Assessment* (pp. 69–119). Academic Press.

Tajfel, H., Billig, M. G., Bundy, R. P., & Flament, C. (1971). Social categorization and intergroup behaviour. *European Journal of Social Psychology, 1*(2), 149–178.

Tajfel, H., & Turner, J. C. (1986). The social identity theory of intergroup behaviour. In S. Worchel & W. G. Austin Eds., *The psychology of intergroup relations* (pp. 7–24). Nelson-Hall.

Taylor, C. (1991). *The malaise of modernity.* House of Anansi.

Totman, R. (1979). *Social causes of illness.* Souvenir.

Wartofsky, M. W. (1982). Piaget's genetic epistemology and the Marxist theory of knowledge. *Revue Internationale de Philosophie, 36*(4), 470–507.

Weiss, G., & Haber, H. F. (Eds.). (1999). *Perspectives on embodiment. Intersections of nature and culture.* Routledge.

Wiesel Commission (2004). *International commission on the Holocaust in Romania.* Final Report_1.p65 (inshr-ew.ro) Retrieved 30 May 2024.

Wong, W. (2009). Retracing the footsteps of Wilhelm Wundt: Explorations in the disciplinary frontiers of psychology and in *Völkerpsychologie. History of Psychology, 12*(4), 229–265.

CHAPTER 3

Development of Social Representation Theory

Since the introduction of social representation theory in the 1950s, it has attracted sustained discussion, leading to developments in theory. In addition, from the outset, researchers have used a range of different research designs, including both quantitative and qualitative methods. It all depended on the topic under investigation and the particular approach within social representation theory. A feature of social representation research is the desire to explore the diversity of perspectives rather than a single uniform perspective. As such, qualitative methods have proved particularly suited to exploring this diversity. In this chapter, we review the basic principles of social representation theory, its developments, and connections with other theories. We also consider the methods used in the original studies and the various qualitative methods that have been introduced in some subsequent studies.

3.1 Basic Concepts

Social representations theory is concerned with how a community or society makes sense of its world. It is not an individual cognitive process but rather a dynamic social and cognitive process. Two perspectives are contained within this definition of social representations. Social representations theory distinguishes between social representations as entities and processes. On the one hand, they are social representations of our everyday

M. Murray, *Social Representations, Health and Illness*,
https://doi.org/10.1007/978-3-031-98494-5_3

reality, and on the other, they are being formed through everyday social interaction. This developmental process is one that occurs through various forms of communication. Thus, research into social representations takes account of both their character and how they evolve. The shared nature of the social representation enables the members of a collective to have a shared understanding of their world and to participate collectively in it.

From the outset, Moscovici was keen to distinguish social representations from other concepts such as attitudes and opinions. In the introduction to the second edition of his classic work, he wrote: 'We do not consider them to be "opinions about" or "images of"; we consider them to be *sui generis* "theories" or "collective sciences" to be used for the interpretation and shaping of the real' (Moscovici, [1976] 2008, p. 10). As theories, they are not simply a classification scheme but a process such that information 'is subject to the work of transformation and evolution that allows it to become a piece of knowledge that most of us will use in our daily lives' (p. 10). This process of transforming information is a social process that occurs in everyday social interaction.

As such, social representations can be considered as both static and dynamic. The static perspective considers them as a network of beliefs, attitudes and behaviours that form the basis of common sense. The focus of the representation is that object which is evaluated and constructed through the social representation. It is a representation of something. The social and dynamic perspective is concerned with how the social representation is constructed through everyday social interaction. It is the act of social representing. Moscovici placed importance on the process of communication in the construction of social representations, which asserts their socially dynamic quality. As he said:

> the word social was meant to indicate that representations are the outcome of an unceasing babble and a permanent dialogue between individuals, a dialogue that is both internal and external, during which individual representations are echoed or complemented (Moscovici, 1984a, p. 950).

Social representations develop in everyday social interaction. Figure 3.1 presents Moscovici's (1984a) semiotic triangle, which is a diagrammatic representation of the process of developing social representations. On the bottom left of the triangular model is the Subject, or person, who is actively engaged with the Alter, or other person, in constructing a social

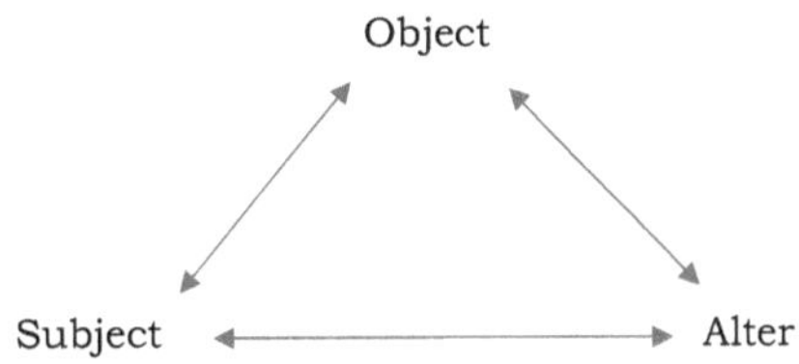

Fig. 3.1 The Ego-Alter-Object triad. Adapted from Marková (2003, p. 152)

representation of the Object. Thus, the Subject (or Ego) and the Alter are involved in an ongoing process of communication about the Object. This communication can take the form of conversation, argument, reading, listening, etc. It is a process that is influenced by social context, history, emotions and ethics. This emphasis on communication is why Moscovici ([1976] 2008) emphasized that 'communication in some sense moulds the very structure of representations' (p. 31).

In this model, the Subject develops knowledge of the Object through social interaction with the Other (Alter). This is not a one-way process; rather, the Subject brings to the encounter particular beliefs and experiences and, through interaction with the Other, grasps the Object. Moscovici (1998a) also emphasized that he was most interested in the process of developing social representations, not simply in the representations themselves.

The process of developing a social representation especially occurs when the person(s) is confronted by an external threat, something that requires understanding in order to take action. This process takes place within a particular socio-cultural context. It also takes place within a temporal/historical context. It was for this reason that Bauer and Gaskell (1999) added time to the triadic model to develop what they described as a 'Toblerone' model of the development of social representations. This expanded model considers the role of past and future elements in the construction of social representations. The triad is immersed in history, coupled with future prospects.

A related concept is that of 'collective remembering', whereby a community or a society has a shared understanding of its history. This collective remembering is carried in its social representations and shapes its present (Wagoner, 2015). This is similar to the idea of the shared narrative, which can be both backward and forward-looking. It can contain stories of past injustices but also of future glories (Selbin, 2010).

Social representations not only enable the social construction of reality but also shape our everyday practices. Moscovici ([1976] 2008) described their function as being 'to shape inter-individual behaviours and communication' (p. *xxx*). This process functions first by 'relating them to a system of values, notions, and practices that enables individuals to orient themselves within the social and material environment, and to master it' (p. *xxxi*). It functions secondly by 'furnishing members of a community with a medium of exchange and a code that allows them to name and classify clearly the various parts of their world and their individual or collective history' (p. *xxxi*).

Further, Moscovici ([1976] 2008) described a social representation as a 'preparation for action'. More specifically:

> it is so not only to the extent that it governs behaviour but above all to the extent that it remodels and reconstitutes the elements of the environment in which the behaviour takes place. It succeeds in giving meaning to behaviour, and in integrating it into a network of relations in which it is bound up with its object. At the same time, it supplies the notions, theories and stocks of observation which render those relations stable and efficacious (p. 9).

Processes: Moscovici posited two important processes that are involved in the development of social representations. The first is *objectification*, through which abstract concepts are given more intelligible substance by objectifying them in a more concrete entity. Moscovici ([1976] 2008) described it as '[the] reabsorbing surplus significations by making them material (and distancing ourselves from them). It also means transferring something that was no more than an inference or symbol to the level of observation' (p. 55). He gave, as an example, how the psychoanalytic terms 'repression' and 'complex' were transformed from abstract scientific concepts into 'manifestations of the real' in everyday language. 'Ideas are no longer perceived to be products of the intellectual activity of certain minds, and are seen as something that exists outside' (p. 55).

This process of objectification takes place through language in everyday communication. Moscovici argued that objectification occurs through three components: *information, figurative schema* and *naturalization*. The first component is *information*, which refers to the details about the external world that the person selects and acts upon. The *figurative schema* is the process whereby the individual processes this information, while *naturalization* is the process whereby these details are given substance (see Marková, 2023, pp. 59–61). Furthermore, there are two processes connecting these components. First, there is the process of selecting information based on the person's values and other social representations. Then, this representation is transformed into social reality—it becomes the reality that the person acts upon.

The second process is *anchoring*, which connects the perception of new phenomena to something more established. It is the process of making something unfamiliar familiar through this connection. As Moscovici ([1976] 2008) explained: 'Society uses the process of anchoring to change a social object into an instrument it can use, and to insert that object into existing social relations on a preferential basis' (p. 104). It is the process by which new, strange ideas are given meaning by connecting them with something that is more familiar. Thus, Freud's idea of the unconscious is given meaning in a Catholic community by connecting it with the idea of conscience, with which its adherents are more familiar. This process is not an individual cognitive process but rather a social process shared by the group. It transforms the object into 'an instrument it can use' (p. 194).

Moscovici ([1976] 2008) distinguished between these two processes: 'To cut a long story short, objectification transposes science into the domain of *being*, and anchoring defines it with the domain of *doing* so as to get around the taboo of communications' (p. 104). Objectification is the content aspect of social representations, while anchoring is the process. It is the use value of anchoring that is of importance. It enables us to act upon the world in a certain way. Considering psychoanalysis, Moscovici ([1976] 2008) described how, through anchoring, it 'becomes a system of interpretation and mutates into a language that allows those problems to be communicated. At this stage, it ceases to be "what we talk about" and becomes "what we use to talk"' (p. 105).

Marková (2023), in her detailed analysis of the different editions of *Psychoanalysis*, makes the point that although in the first edition Moscovici placed objectification first and anchoring second, in the second edition this order is reversed. This is an important distinction, as it emphasizes that in the first edition the process of objectification is the innovative one, which creates something new and then anchors the phenomenon among related characteristics. In the second edition, the emphasis is given to anchoring, which gives less importance to the process of objectification.

A dialectical and dialogical (language-based) perspective overcomes the dispute regarding the sequence of these processes. Rather, it is an ongoing interactive process or spiral, or in Hegelian terms, 'a circle returning within itself'. Thus, while it may not be possible to discern the sequence, it is through the ongoing interaction of these processes that social representations develop. Marková added that 'individuals and groups may shift their meanings, going forwards and backwards depending on changes in their experiencing of the socio-cultural and political environment' (Marková, 2023, pp. 92–93). Thus, the process occurs not in a vacuum but within a particular socio-historic context.

Cognitive polyphasia: From the outset, Moscovici was aware of contradictions in the content of social representations. They could contain contradictions in the sense that certain forms of knowledge may be more dominant at certain times and in certain situations. Moscovici ([1976] 2008, p. 191) introduced the term *cognitive polyphasia* to describe how people can hold apparently contradictory ideas. He later extended this idea to argue that 'knowledge is polyphasic and (that) people in fact have different representations depending on to which group they belong, the profession they exercise, and so on' (Moscovici & Marková, 1998, p. 385).

Cognitive polyphasia concerns the different representations of a phenomenon that can be held by a community and which become apparent in different contexts. Thus, rather than having a fixed social representation of a phenomenon, a community can have a more fluid representation, but one which is constrained by the social context. The community is constantly engaged in the process of making sense of a changing world. It is aware of different and even contradictory representations which are presented in everyday social communication.

When he introduced this concept originally, Moscovici described it as a hypothesis that required further research. It does not concern the existence of different ways of thinking, which are present in different situations. Rather, it concerns the simultaneous presence of different ways of thinking, leading to certain tensions. There is not a feeling of equilibrium and accommodation of contrary positions, but instead a state of ongoing disputation. As Moscovici ([1976], 2008) argued:

> In a global manner one can say that the dynamic coexistence – interference or specialization – of the distinct modalities of knowledge, corresponding to definite relations between man (sic) and his environment, *determines a state of cognitive polyphasia*. This hypothesis prompts us to broaden our

> perspectives. Cognitive systems should be construed as developing systems and not uniquely as systems tending to equilibrium. Operative or formal judgements habitually represent one of these dominant terms in a field of personal or group preoccupations, while playing a subordinate role elsewhere. (p. 190–191).

Marková (2023) argued that objectification and anchoring, along with cognitive polyphasia, are unique to Moscovici's conception of social representation and place it as clearly different from Durkheim's collective representations. The former is dynamic and exists only through interdependence with humans who create these concepts and the ensuing social phenomena (p. 98). The latter exists independently of social interaction. Indeed, Marková (2003) emphasized that, from her perspective, 'none of the fundamental concepts in the social representations of *Psychoanalysis* derive from Durkheim' (p. 87).

In an earlier conversation with Marková, Moscovici commented that it was via Piaget that he began to grasp the ideas of Durkheim. He said: 'I really started to read the fathers of this idea (representation), Durkheim and Lévy-Bruhl, in the 1980s [. . .]. After all, Piaget (1932) took this concept, and many other theoretical issues about which he wrote in the early part of his book on moral judgement, from Durkheim. So in a way I took Durkheim's heritage without being aware of it' (Moscovici & Marková, 1998, p. 395). However, in adopting Durkheim's model of representations, Moscovici transformed it into a socially dynamic phenomenon.

This socially dynamic characteristic was one that was commended in a Marxist critique by Alain Baubion-Broye et al. (1977) who preferred Moscovici's social representations to Durkheim's collective representations. Although Durkheim's conception of representation was of a fixed collection of beliefs that shaped relations between humans, Moscovici's conception was a dynamic conception of representations that provided a guide for social action. As Baubion-Broye et al. argued, the social representation:

> is not a given which is imposed on individuals but an act, all the more difficult to execute, as it embraces diverse perspectives. This remark opposes RS [social representation] to 'collective representation' as Durkheim understands it: as a totality of obligatory beliefs, which organizes the field of relationships to be established between the various

> aspects of reality, and the value that must be attributed to them. On the contrary, we hypothesize that RS is constructed, in the communications that are established between the individuals of a group, by means of denials, that is to say, judgments assumed by the subjects in an effort to consciously define a perspective of action[1](Baubion-Broye et al., 1977, p. 51, trans.).

Thus, while social representations can impose themselves upon the group or community, they can also orient the group towards change.

Themata: A concept that further develops this socially dynamic characteristic of social representations is *themata*. This concerns what Moscovici and Vignaux (1994/2000) have described as 'source ideas' (p. 177), which lie 'at the heart of social representations'. This concept was initially developed by the physicist Holton (1978), who defined themata as 'oppositional antinomies', which can describe the character of scientific concepts (p. ix). Holton referred specifically to Piaget's concepts of accommodation and assimilation as examples of themata (Marková, 2003, p. 183). Moscovici and Vignaux added that they...

> bring about the generation of axiomatics [taken for granted phenomena] in the evolution of our representations of the world. They take the form of 'notions', that is to say, of 'potential places' of meaning as generators of conceptions, they are 'virtual' because these 'places' can only be characterised through discourse, through justifications and arguments which 'nurture' them in the form of productions of meanings (p. 177).

They also defined them in terms of '*systems of oppositions* (i.e. terms which are contrasted in order to be related)' (p. 179).

This led them to present a 'configurational system', which placed themata as playing a central 'generative function' in the development of social representations. These themata proceed through the processes of anchoring and objectification to the development of laws and rules, which

[1] 'elle n'est pas un donne, qui s'impose aux individus, mais un acte, d'autant plus difficile à executer qu'il embrasse davantage d'objectifs divergents. Cette remarque oppose la RS à la « représentation collective » telle que Durkheim l'entend: comme un ensemble de croyances obligatoires, qui organise le champ des relations à établir entre les différents aspects de la réalité, et la valeur qui doit leur être attribuée. Au contraire, nous émettons l'hypothèse que la RS se construit, dans les communications qui s'établissent entre les individus d'un groupe, au moyen de dénégations, c'est-à-dire de jugements assumés par les sujets dans le but de définir consciemment une perspective d'action.'

enable us to make sense of the world. However, these themata are not always clearly evident: '"Themata" never reveal themselves clearly; not even part of them is definitely attainable, so much are they intricately interwoven within a certain collective memory inscribed in language' (p. 182). These themata are deeply embedded in a culture, and we draw upon them in everyday social interaction.

Marková (2023) has further refined our understanding of themata, describing them as 'antithetical or dialectical oppositions', which can be dormant. While antinomies are widespread in diverse belief systems, they can become themata 'if, in the course of certain social and historical events, e.g., political, economic, religious and so on, they turn into problems and become the focus of social attention and a source of tension and conflict' (Marková, 2003, p. 184). It is then that they become involved in the generation of social representations.

Communication of social representations: Although social representations may develop within a particular group at a particular time, they also spread. It is for this reason that Moscovici spent considerable effort detailing how these representations spread. The first communication process is *diffusion,* whereby a variety of ideas are circulated in society via the media and other means. These ideas are not formally organized and it gives the opportunity for the receiver to explore a variety of discordant views. Moscovici identified three features of diffusion: it is concrete, attractive and rapid (Moscovici, [1976] Moscovici, 2008, p. 216). These features of the media are effective because they engage the reader and attract readership. In some cases, the media can use humour and irony as a way of distancing the publication from the message—it's just a joke. Thus, the message is concealed or not made explicit.

Then there is the more organized format of spreading ideas. Moscovici distinguished between *propaganda* and *propagation*—the former being more direct attempts to transform public ideas. Propaganda was described as a deliberate effort to convey a particular viewpoint and to denigrate contrary perspectives. The aim is to convince the receiver of the validity of its approach. It was more common in the press with an obvious ideological perspective, such as that of the Communist Party, but was also apparent in the press associated with the Catholic Church. Moscovici referred to Lenin (1902), who had considered the importance of propaganda in his pamphlet *What Is to Be Done.* Lenin saw propaganda as a means of: a) shaping a group's worldview, b) promoting an awareness of the group's individuality and integration into society and c) complementing other forms of communication and social action. Moscovici ([1976] 2008) noted that Lenin's writings 'abound with psychological insights and practical recommendations, but they do not give rise to any deeper conceptual systematisation' (p. 285), which he sought to develop.

At that time, there was intense interest in the psychology of propaganda. During the war, Joseph Goebbels had been head of the Nazi Ministry of Public Enlightenment and Propaganda and very much admired the ideas on crowd psychology developed by Gustave Le Bon (1841–1931). Moscovici (1985) explored these ideas later in his discussion of crowd psychology. In Britain, the Ministry of Information had used various propaganda techniques during the war (e.g., Whyte, 2018). George Orwell had worked in that ministry and possibly used the experience subsequently in writing his classic novel *1984.* In France, after the war, Charles de Gaulle appointed the novelist André Malraux (1901–1976) as the Minister of Culture. His remit was to promote the arts throughout French society and thus reassert what was seen as a weakening of French society due to low-level popular culture and urban life. It was this low-level culture that had supposedly contributed to the fall in French morale and the nation's collapse in the face of the Nazi onslaught (Hewitt, 2003). Moscovici ([1976] 2008) described propaganda as 'one of the obsessions of the age', reflecting 'the fear that individuals might lapse into dependency' (p. 284) as a result of the post-war political turmoil.

He went on to identify two functions of propaganda. The first, he described as *regulation,* whereby the group asserts its identity as distinct from any neighbouring groups, and the second is *organization*, whereby the aim is to transform the perceived content of the social field. He argued that both functions become more pronounced at times of crisis (*a polarized situation*).

Propaganda is not, however, a singular transmission of a particular viewpoint. Rather, the audience must be convinced that the message is correct. An amusing example of this process is the story of the East German resident visiting the West after the fall of the Berlin Wall. Looking at the content of the media, she commented on the widespread nature of pro-Western propaganda. The West German resident was surprised at this description of the media and retorted that there was surely similar pro-government propaganda in the East. The East German resident agreed but added that they didn't believe in it (see Erpenbeck, 2023).

Propagation is more indirect, as was reflected in the newspapers that presented a Catholic viewpoint, investigated by Moscovici ([1976] 2008). In this case, the authority was divided in its views of psychoanalysis. The newspapers attempted to present some commonalities between the Catholic faith and psychoanalysis, but they did not insist on unanimity. Their aim was to directly challenge the new framework (psychoanalysis) while integrating it into an existing framework.

Although these different processes are more often associated with certain organized groups, this is not to say that they are unique to those groups. Thus, although the communist press may emphasize the propaganda, it could also introduce aspects of diffusion and propaganda as a means of attracting a broader audience and even concealing its more deliberate message.

A central feature in these different forms of communication was the power differential between those conveying and those receiving the information. As Moscovici ([1976] 2008) said:

> The diffusion of a science is valuable because it is informative, but anyone who is in possession of knowledge is also in possession of power. He is competent and dominant; he is an expert and not just a sender, and the other is no longer just a receiver, but a layman (p. 48).

This is somewhat similar to Michel Foucault's argument around power-knowledge (*le pouvoir-savoir*). He argued that power is based on knowledge and makes use of knowledge. Furthermore, claims to knowledge by one group can enable their power over another group (Foucault, 2020).

Moscovici also distinguished between the *reified* and the *consensual* universe. While scientific knowledge is the property of the reified universe, common sense knowledge belongs to the consensual universe. Knowledge in the reified universe aims towards an impartial explanation of the world. Knowledge in the consensual universe is more variable and, as Marková summarizes 'thrives on negotiation and mutual acceptance' (Moscovici & Marková, 1998, p. 386). Furthermore, scientific knowledge proceeds by systematic reasoning with a focus on supposedly established facts. Conversely, common sense is based upon consensus and collective memory. However, both kinds of knowledge are based upon reason. As Moscovici (1998b) said: "All representations are rational, even if, to paraphrase Orwell, some appear more rational than others" (p. 416). Thus, there are different ways of being rational, even if the scientific sense is the dominant one, such that common sense is often derided as being irrational. However, the distinction between these two universes is not always clear-cut, such that social representations can draw from both.

Types of social representation: Social representation theory is concerned not just with a phenomenon that exists but also with how it develops and transforms. While this social representation takes place in everyday communication, it is subject to the status and power of the participants. Moscovici (1984b) emphasized the importance of the socio-political context in understanding the transformation of social representations. He referred to three types of social representation:

a. *Hegemonic* representations are those shared by members of a structured group but have not been produced by the group; rather, they have been imposed upon it and are resistant to change.
b. *Polemical* representations are those that develop during periods of social conflict, are produced by different groups in society, and reflect antagonistic relations.
c. *Emancipated* representations emerge in the circulation of knowledge between groups and are accepted as different forms of social knowledge.

The hegemonic representations are reified in the sense that they are stable and resistant to change. In that sense, they are similar to Durkheim's collective representations. Conversely, the polemical and emancipated representations are subject to change and can be considered dialogical. The polemical representations are based upon the form of communication typified by Moscovici as propaganda and strive to become hegemonic. Emancipated representations are based upon Piagetian mutual respect and cooperation and are subject to change through open dialogue. A central part of this change is doubt, whereby beliefs can be subject to challenge.

3.2 Theoretical Developments

Over the past 60 years, there have been various developments in social representation theory. These developments were welcomed by Moscovici and will be considered briefly here.

Socio-cultural: This approach emphasizes that the focus and method of social representation research are socially and culturally located. From the outset, Moscovici had stressed the need for social psychology to connect with anthropology and even argued that 'social psychology should be a kind of anthropology of our culture' (Moscovici & Marková, 1998, p. 409). Both Herzlich (1973) and Jodelet (1991) developed this approach in their studies of health and madness. Since then, other researchers have considered the importance of the social and cultural context of social representations.

Marková (2023) characterized this approach in terms of three characteristics. The first is the interdependence between the inner world of groups and individuals and other outer worlds. These take place within particular social and cultural contexts and are thus unique to those settings. The second feature of this approach is the concern with the imagined world. Thus, researchers adopting this approach often explore the role of images in social representations. An early example is the work of de Rosa (1987) in her study of the images of madness in history. The third feature is the role of collective memory and myths. These historical phenomena influence the content and organization of social representations. An example is the work by de Saint-Laurent (2018), which explored how grand political plots from the French Revolution continue to pervade contemporary French parliamentary debates.

Jodelet (2012a) also proposed an analytical model of social representations, as displayed in Fig. 3.2. She argued that they operate within three spheres of belonging. The first is the *trans-subjective* sphere, which refers

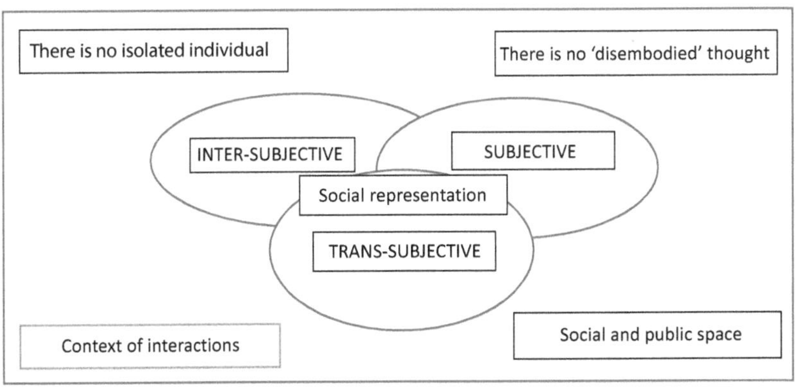

Fig. 3.2 Spheres of belonging in social representations. Adapted from Jodelet (2012a)

to the social and public space within which social representations circulate. The *inter-subjective* sphere is concerned with the situation in which social representations are established through dialog and communication. Finally, there is the *subjective* sphere, which is concerned with the processes by which one becomes involved in the construction or acceptance of social representations. This process occurs within a bodily self, is both cognitive and emotional, and depends upon experience in the world.

Socio-genetic: This approach is concerned with the development of social representations through social interaction. Marková (2023) traced this approach to the work of Doise and his colleagues, who noted how children performed spatial representation tasks better in pairs than alone. He and his colleagues developed the idea of socio-genetic conflict as being the basis of children's cognitive development (Doise & Mugny, 1975). Subsequently, Gerard Duveen (1951–2008) argued that the child's understanding of the world develops in social interaction, as in the Subject-Alter-Object triad (Duveen, 2001a). He explored how children's explanations of moral arguments depended upon whether they were alone or with others.

The development of social representations is an ongoing process as new phenomena emerge in society. Duveen and Lloyd (2007) argued that there are three types of transformation in the development of social representations: the *sociogenetic,* which is concerned with the construction and transformation of social representations about certain phenomena within social groups; the *ontogenetic,* which is concerned with the development of individuals with reference to these social representations; and the *microgenetic*, which is concerned with how the social representations evolve in everyday social interaction. At the sociogenetic level, there is a concern with how media and other representations are transformed within social groups. At the ontogenetic level, a longitudinal study design is preferred to explore how social representations are enacted as individuals develop. At the microgenetic level, the focus is on everyday conversation, which is apparent in interviews and ethnography as well as surveys and experiments. The diary questionnaire and the interviews were at the microgenetic level, while the media analysis was at the sociogenetic level. Thus, from the outset, social representation researchers were keen to use qualitative methods, although they became more sophisticated over time.

Structural: This approach was developed by Jean-Claude Abric (1941–2012) from Aix-en-Provence. He argued that social representations have a certain internal organization with a central core and various peripheral elements (Abric, 2001). To explore this further, Abric conducted research into how words and concepts were associated in discussions about certain topics. He was interested in what he described as the hierarchical structure of these concepts. The central core was considered to be the stable collection of the most influential concepts. It has a generating and organizing function in that it generates the overall meaning of the representation and organizes the internal relationship between elements. The central core was stable and not dependent on the social context. Conversely, the peripheral elements were more variable and depended upon the social context. They protect the central core by their flexibility in providing justifications for apparent contradictions.

Organizing principles: This approach was developed by Willem Doise and his group at the University of Geneva. According to them, social representations can be characterized as 'organising principles of differences in individual positioning' (Doise et al., 1993: 154). They are 'reference points in relation to which individuals position themselves according to specific social experiences they share with other individuals' (p. 155). They make the point that consensus in beliefs is not an essential characteristic of social representations. Rather, 'they may result in different or even opposed positions taken by individuals in relation to common reference points' (Doise et al., 1993, p. 4). It is the shared reference points that are essential, from which individuals and groups orient themselves.

Doise (1986) also considered the different levels of explanation in social psychology. There are four primary levels. The *intrapsychic* level is concerned with psychological phenomena, such as attitudes and personality, which are used to explain social behaviour. Then there is the *interpersonal* level, which focuses on the interaction between people within a certain situation. The *positional* level expands the interpersonal level to consider the differences in social position between the individuals concerned. Finally, there is the *ideological* level, which is concerned with the system of beliefs and representations that validate a particular social order. This ideological level is constituted through various social representations. This approach has encouraged researchers to deliberately explore multiple levels of explanation of different phenomena (e.g., Murray, 2000).

Dialogical: An approach that has attracted increasing interest is that developed by Marková (2003, 2023). For years, she had been applying dialectical concepts to an understanding of interpersonal communication and to developing an alternative to what she described as the Cartesian approach within psychology. By the 1990s, she began to investigate its potential value in exploring the dynamics of social representations.

She argued that communication is an implicit aspect of social representations and took this up in her conversation with Moscovici (Moscovici & Marková, 2000) where he argued that 'one conditions the other because we cannot communicate unless we share certain representations, and a representation is shared and enters our social heritage when it becomes an object of interest and of communication' (p. 274). This dialectical approach to the study of communication, Marková (2003) termed dialogical. The emphasis of this approach is that the Alter always intervenes in the interaction of the Subject with the Object.

3.3 Links with Other Theories

There have been various attempts to connect social representation theory with other social psychological theories. With the growth of different psychological approaches to understanding how we make sense of the world, it is sometimes difficult to distinguish one from another. Let us consider some of these related approaches.

Social cognition: This is the dominant approach within contemporary social psychology and is concerned with the cognitive processes involved in making sense of the world. A key example of this approach is attribution theory, which was developed by Fritz Heider (1958). He was keen to systematize how the lay person attributes causes for events in the social world. He conceived of the lay person as a 'naïve scientist' who could make errors in their assessment of events. Thus, attribution theorists were often concerned with attribution biases and errors, although they largely neglected the broader socio-cultural context. The social cognition approach has had great influence within health psychology, where the use of such approaches as the Theory of Reasoned Action (Fishbein & Ajzen, 1975) and Self-Regulation Theory (Leventhal et al., 1980) is extensive. Some researchers (e.g., Augoustinos, 2001) have explored connections between the two theories. However, the general focus of social cognition is more on individual cognitive processing rather than on the dynamic interaction between the individual and society.

Discursive psychology: This approach focuses on the study of naturally occurring discourse, which is considered a form of social action (Edwards & Potter, 1992). The detailed study of discourse promoted by this approach can contribute to exploring how social representations are negotiated in everyday social interaction. However, the singular focus on discourse ignores the broader cultural context within which discourse occurs. As Susana Batel and Paula Castro (2019) stress, 'meanings are constructed and negotiated in the interplay between the microprocesses of interaction [. . .] and the macroprocesses of institutional and cultural practices' (p. 430). There remain other theoretical tensions. From the outset, Potter and Wetherell (Potter & Wetherell, 1987) dismissed social representation theory as being saddled with 'a weight of unformulated cognitive baggage' (p. 146). They and subsequent discursive critics have characterized social representations as solely cognitive or mental entities.

Batel and Castro (2018, 2019) have explored this and other criticisms. One problem is that different versions of social representation theory have placed varying emphasis on the importance of communication. The weak version places more emphasis on cognition, whereas the strong version places more emphasis on communication. Thus, discursive psychology critics have focused on the weak version, such as Abric's structural approach, and neglected the strong version, which emphasizes the importance of communication. Furthermore, they assume a limited version of cognition as existing solely in the heads of individuals, rather than being generated through social interaction and culture. The discursive approach also argues that social representations are not concerned with action, but from a more critical stance, representation is action. Social representations are practical knowledge that is used in social interaction. As Caroline Howarth (2006) emphasized: 'We could say that representations can be "used" to defend and sustain a particular construction of reality, or "mentioned" in resistance to another version of reality' (p. 68).

Narrative: Narrative psychology is an approach that developed especially in North America in the 1980s with a series of influential publications (e.g. Sarbin, 1986). It argued that people are natural storytellers and explain the world through different types of stories. In his original study, Moscovici ([1976] 2008) did refer to the narrative content of everyday communication.

> Effectively a social representation condenses a quite direct, diversified and diffuse collective reflection, each of its participants being up to a point an autodidact, and like every autodidact takes both the dictionary and the encyclopaedia as an ideal. Hence the narrative, descriptive, arborescent style, with its repetitions and its goings and comings between 'texts' produced by 'thoughts used for immediate communication' (p. 31).

Later, he observed in his study of psychoanalysis the expansive nature of storytelling: '"Stories" are embellished with jokes or funny anecdotes [. . .] creating a density around the object [. . .] and giving it a "spoken' reality"' (p. 47).

Subsequently, several researchers began to study the value of this approach in exploring both the content and dynamics of social representations. László (1997) argued that narrative underlies the structure of social representations. He noted the narrative content of the interviews conducted in the studies by Herzlich (1973). Murray (1997, 2002, 2024) remarked not only on the use of narratives in the construction of social representations but also on the narrative structure of social representations, comparing them with collective narratives.

Other researchers took up this idea. For example, Jovchelovitch (2007) stressed that 'it is by telling stories that social knowledge comes to life, and with it, the representation of the past, and the presentation of identity' (p. 82). Furthermore, Jovchelovitch and Bauer (2000) promoted the use of the narrative interview as a means of collecting information about a particular topic. They stressed the importance of considering the socio-historical context within which the narrative is embedded. Flick (2000a) developed a technique known as the *episodic interview*, which provided participants with the opportunity to develop narrative accounts of their world. Flick also developed the concept of *retrospective anchoring* to describe how people refer to previous events in their interpretations of the world.

Social identity: Social identity theory is concerned with how people define themselves with reference to others. This approach was initiated by Tajfel and further developed by John Turner and others (Tajfel, 1978; Tajfel & Turner, 1986). The basic social identity approach argues that our identity is created through our membership in a social group and how it defines itself with reference to the in-group and as distinct from the out-group. In doing so, the person strives to maintain and enhance a positive social identity.

Social representations are intimately connected with social identities. These identities are not just of small social groups but of much larger collectives. Groups are defined through their shared social representations. Reflecting on this process, Moscovici (1998a) noted that 'the ideas and beliefs that enable people to live are incarnated in specific structures (clans, churches, social movements, families, clubs, etc.) and adopted by the individuals who are a part of them' (p. 216).

Several researchers have explored empirically the connections between social identity and social representation theory. Howarth (2007) argued that these theories are two sides of the same coin. Specifically, 'in positioning ourselves in relation to others—that is, in asserting, performing or *doing* identity—we reveal our perspective on the world and our ways of seeing and constructing the world, or our social representations' (p. 133). She went on to explore how children from a community in London perceived others from different ethnic backgrounds. Using storytelling and drawings, she explored the different ways these children represented 'race'. She identified three dominant ways of representing 'race': as real, as imposed, and as contested. She found that the children 'used all three representations to different degrees in positioning themselves in the racialized relations of inclusion and friendship at school' (p. 139). She placed these representations within the socio-political context and concluded that not only are these social representations of race/ethnicity intimately connected with social identity, but they 'are anchored in histories of white privilege, oppression, and violence' (p. 151).

Othering is part of the process of ingroup-outgroup differentiation with associated power dynamics. 'Othering typically necessitates the distillation of social identities into distinct classifications: the majority ingroup who embody hegemonic normativity and minority outgroups who may personify alien (and thus potentially subversive) identities' (Bhugra et al., 2023, p. 235). This can lead to exclusion and rejection of the outgroup. However, this is not automatic. Rather, different forms of thinking can lead to inclusion rather than exclusion. Moscovici (2002) distinguished between two forms of thinking for representing otherness: stigmatic, which leads to inferiority, and symbolic thinking, which recognizes the difference but not in a negative sense. Or, as the American writer Audre Lord (1934–1992) said: 'It is not our differences that divide us. It is our inability to recognise, accept and celebrate those differences' (Lord, 1986). A study of the social representations of undernourished children held by mothers in Nepal found that the type of othering was related to the different forms of thinking about undernutrition (Caillaud et al., 2024).

Phenomenology: Phenomenology is concerned with understanding lived experiences. Merleau-Ponty emphasized the importance of understanding the role of human perception in everyday life. Marková (2023: 41–42) detailed three aspects of Merleau-Ponty's work that influenced Moscovici's thinking: 1. Life experience was an open and dynamic system such that representation is not separate but connected to the lived experience. 2. The living body embraced the whole of an individual's sense-making by perception and speaking. 3. Perception is of primary importance in understanding experience. For Merleau-Ponty these processes were individual, whereas for Moscovici they were a social psychological process and developed through social interaction. He argued that his interest in social representations 'has always been in them in the making, not as already made' (p. 394). The body is central to Merleau-Ponty's phenomenology. He argued that you cannot separate the mind from the body, and knowledge is intrinsically related to our bodily experiences.

Other philosophers have continued the discussion of the nature of representations in phenomenology. Heidegger introduced the concept *of Dasein*, which is concerned with those aspects of existence of which one is not conscious. Charles Taylor (2016) took up this perspective and argued against the primacy of representations in our interpretation of the world. Instead, he argued that behind these representations is an unarticulated background. Taylor was developing what he described as a philosophical anthropology. The problem lies in exploring this unarticulated background, how it develops, and how it can be investigated.

Psychodynamic: Since the focus of Moscovici's original research was on social representations of psychoanalysis, it is not surprising that this approach has many connections. Primarily, Moscovici was interested in how psychoanalysis was represented in the media and in everyday conversation. Moscovici had a continuing interest in psychoanalysis and even described the unconscious as 'the most significant discovery in the history of psychology' (Moscovici, 1993a, p. 48). In his own research, he found that the four most well-known psychoanalytic terms were complex, repression, unconscious/subconscious and libido. Moscovici suggested that the continued dominance of these traditional psychoanalytic concepts, despite further theoretical refinement of psychoanalysis, was because 'the image of psychoanalysis initially crystallized around certain notions which could not then be rejected' (p. 62). These notions had developed in French society over one or two generations and were resistant to change.

Other researchers have referred to hidden emotional processes as underlying social representations. Jodelet (1991), in her study of a community's understanding of mental illness, suggested that their fears of the illness were linked with folk fantasizes and superstition. In our work on cancer, popular fear of the disease was linked with ancient ideas of malevolence and contagion (Murray & McMillan, 1993). Joffe (1996) has explored the potential of repression as a mediating process in social representations of HIV/AIDS.

Critical and cultural studies: Critical social psychology challenges the dominant, disinterested positivist stance of mainstream social psychology. Instead, it considers the ideological forces shaping both the theory and methods of the discipline. It draws upon ideas from various critical theories, such as Marxism, feminism, social constructionism, etc., to develop a more critical understanding of social relationships, social practices and society, and considers how the discipline can contribute to broader human emancipation (Gough et al., 2013; Midlands Psychology Group, 2022).

A particular focus in critical psychology has been that of power and powerlessness. Although Moscovici did not explicitly address the issue of power, he did refer to it in his later writings, where he noted that 'there is a power of ideas that makes itself felt in its highest form when representations acquire the intensity of a belief' (Moscovici, 1988, p. 230).

A key figure in the development of critical theory has been Michel Foucault (1926–1984). His classic work *Folie et Déraison: Histoire de la Folie à l'âge classique* (Foucault, 1961/1965) was published in the same year as the first edition of Moscovici's classic work (Moscovici, 1961). In his second edition, Moscovici ([1976] 2008) does make reference to this work in his discussion on the boundaries between the normal and the pathological. However, he does not refer to Foucault's archaeological approach or to his ideas on power. Moscovici's approach was more dialectical in that ordinary people were more actively involved in the development and maintenance of representations rather than they being imposed upon them (Vidal-Naquet, 2001).

In developing a critical social representation theory, Howarth et al. (2014) referred to the different types of social representations. They argued that while social representations can attain hegemonic status and support prevailing ideologies, they are also open to change. Social representations 'allow for resistance and change through the active re-appropriation of existing knowledge and identity positions' (p. 20). Polemical representations are those that are engaged in the process of challenging established positions.

Lilian Negura et al. (2019) have used Arendt's (1972) conceptualization of power as making action possible, dependent upon the legitimacy or level of recognition granted by others. In the same way, social representations are prerequisites for action since they contribute to the very construction of reality. Furthermore, since power is dependent upon the legitimacy it is granted, legitimacy itself is dependent upon social representations. Finally, power is made possible by the internalization of these social representations. Negura et al. used Jodelet's (2012a) three levels to further conceptualize the operation of power. At the trans-subjective level, social representations legitimize the power of dominant groups through their anchorage in certain themata, ideologies and social norms. At the inter-subjective level, social representations define the type of communication between individuals and groups, and thus the possibilities for action. Finally, at the subjective level, social representations are involved in the internalization of power relations.

The related field of cultural studies has had a particular concern with how cultural practices are shaped by broader political forces. It is concerned with the operation of political ideology in shaping notions of class, gender, and ethnicity. Although it was developed by Marxists in the 1950s, cultural studies has since broadened its theoretical base to include a much greater range of critical theorists, drawing on ideas from postcolonial studies, semiotics, imagology and other disciplines. The socio-cultural approach to the study of social representations particularly connects with this growing approach.

One area is concerned with how certain phenomena are represented in different arenas and how the public engages with these images. These representations can range from ancient art forms, through classical portrayals in paintings, sculpture and literature, through to contemporary portrayals in photographs, films and the media. Stuart Hall developed a particular theoretical approach to argue that visual images, language, and discourse work as 'systems of representation' (Hall, 1997). Certain representations can attain a dominant position because they possess certain power. Hall (1997) described the practices of representation as 'the embodying of concepts, ideas, and emotions in symbolic form which can be meaningfully interpreted' (p. 10). He further argued that representations enable us to intersubjectively communicate about both the 'real' and the 'fictional' world. This connection has been taken up by social representation researchers (e.g. Winskell, 2021).

The concern with images has been central to the concept of objectification in social representations. It is through this process that we grasp a concrete image of a complex social and biological process. These images can be shared and transferred historically. For example, justice is represented by a woman holding a set of scales. Recently, Cohen et al. (2022)

examined the editorial illustrations posted by French newspapers about COVID-19 on Facebook in 2020. Analysis of these images revealed 12 iconic patterns. The three most common were healthcare workers (mainly a healthcare worker beside a patient in a bed), individuals (usually a person with a sad expression) and ghost towns (empty streets). These images contribute to the objectification of the disease. It is obvious that social representation theory has developed linkages with other social psychological and social scientific theories. Their importance will depend upon the topic of investigation and confirm that there is no singular interpretation of a phenomenon.

3.4 Early Research

One of the strengths of the social representation theory, which is sometimes described as a meta-theory, is its ability to integrate various theoretical and methodological perspectives, e.g., social constructionism, ethogeny and discursive social psychology (Jodelet, 2012b). It can also explore the study of phenomena at different levels—individual, interpersonal, intergroup and ideological (Doise, 1986). Furthermore, it can connect the social sciences with the humanities. Admittedly, this expansive agenda can sometimes appear unwieldy in contrast to many small, limited-variable models that dominate in social psychology.

Research into social representations has been very flexible in its use of methods. This can sometimes be confusing for those who prefer either a quantitative or qualitative approach to research. From the outset, it has used a combination of research methods, although increasingly there has been a preference for different qualitative methods. Moscovici (1998b) cautioned against a search for methodological purity. As he said:

> Methods are only means toward an end. If they become an end or a criterion of the selection of topics and ideas, then they are just another form of professional censorship. So you can call me a methodological opportunist and I will not feel insulted (p. 268).

From the outset, researchers were keen to grasp the development of social representations in everyday communication. As Moscovici argued: 'Communication is part of the study of representations, because representations are generated in this process of communication and then, of course, expressed through language' (Moscovici & Marková, 1998a,

p. 403). It was for this reason that social representation researchers were particularly drawn to a range of more qualitative and ethnographic methods, where they could explore everyday communication.

If we look at the three classic original studies by Moscovici, Herzlich and Jodelet, we can see their early use of qualitative methods. They were less influenced by the quantitative and experimental social psychology. Much later, Apfelbaum (2009) described these French social psychologists as 'a generation without forefathers' (p. 10). The aim of these methods was 'to rehabilitate common knowledge which is guided in our language and in our daily life' (Moscovici & Marková, 1998, p. 375). The three early studies of social representations contain many important lessons for both theory and method. Here, we will briefly consider each of these studies, which are examined in greater detail in subsequent chapters.

Psychoanalysis: In his original study, which was conducted in the 1950s, Moscovici (1967) used three different methods to investigate social representations of psychoanalysis—the notebook-questionnaire, the interview and newspaper analysis. The notebook-questionnaire consisted of a standard questionnaire followed up several days later by an interview. Moscovici described these as free interviews (*entretiens libres*), to which he 'attached as much, if not more, importance as to the questionnaires'. A total of 2,265 participants were interviewed by 'student volunteers who expressed an interest in it'. Most of the participants were residents of Paris, with two small groups living in the provinces (Grenoble and Lyon) (Moscovici, [1976] 2008, p. *xxxiv*). The student and professional participants were interviewed a few days after the questionnaire survey.

The interviews were subsequently coded so that he could consider the relationship between themes and conduct some limited statistical analyses. In his report, he combined the results of the quantitative analysis of the interviews with substantial extracts from them to illustrate particular issues. The media study involved a content analysis of 1640 newspaper articles that mentioned psychoanalysis. These articles were provided by a specialist newspaper cuttings service. Moscovici described his findings as provisional and 'open-ended in that they can provide the basis for analogous work and experiments capable of grasping the processes that have been explored' (p. xxxvii).

The use of the survey–interview was central to his research. In using the interview, he was perhaps influenced by the work of Jean Piaget, whom he had met in Paris. At that time, Piaget was exploring the development of a French version of the intelligence test and worked with children to find out what they thought of the various items. In his work, Piaget engaged children in 'conversations patterned after psychiatric questioning, with the aim of discovering something about the reasoning process under that lying their right, but especially their wrong answer' (Piaget, 1952; in Duveen, 2001b, p. 166). Moscovici (1998b) reflected later that when he came upon Piaget's work, he was almost 30 (about 1955) and 'after I read it I was in a state of shock [...] my thinking liberated itself from innumerable constraining notions with respect both to the methods and to the significant questions that our science addressed' (p. 411).

The free interviews were 'coded in accordance with certain themes and certain categories that allowed me to grasp how they related to one another and to present them in a statistical manner' (Moscovici, [1976] 2008, p. xxxv). Further, he distinguished between 'group-centred' and 'content-centred' coding of the interviews. Using the group-centred coding, it was possible to 'define the group's modalities of expression with regard to a given object'. By this is meant: does the group talk about the object in abstract or concrete terms, and does it have a 'real' or 'ideal' image of it? The content-centred coding was designed to separate out the most frequently occurring themes and then the associations between them. Thus, Moscovici was combining more qualitative with quantitative approaches to his analysis of the interviews. Of particular importance was that he aimed to identify how different categories were related to each other.

Moscovici was cautious and 'placed draconian limitations on the generality of the results [...] until such time as the appropriate methodology comes into being' (p. xxxiii). His work preceded the subsequent discussion about theoretical generalizability (Maxwell & Chmiel, 2014) and although he was using qualitative methods, it was still within a positivist epistemology, admittedly with much latitude. It was much later that he described social representation theory as being social constructionist, but he was working at a time when social psychology was very much asserting its scientific status. Later, Moscovici expressed his frustration with much of experimental research: 'Laboratory experiments could sometimes become no more than a series of little studies, one leading to another, one a refinement of the previous one and so on, altogether a kind of closed intellectual world' (Moscovici & Marková, 2000, p. 167).

He stressed that the findings of his study were 'provisional because of the way they were established and they are open-ended in that they can provide the basis for analogous work and experiments capable of grasping the processes that have been explored'. He continued: 'My desire to explore future possibilities sometimes led me to stray away from conventionally strict empirical doctrine in the hope that I would one day be better equipped to consolidate observations for which there is as yet insufficient evidence' (Moscovici, [1976] 2008, p. xxxvii).

Of particular importance was his content analysis of a sample of newspapers. He analysed a large sample of newspapers, which he classified as having a Communist or Catholic orientation. This enabled him to explore the socio-political and moral context of social representations of psychoanalysis. The Communist press was more likely to emphasize the theoretical or scientific aspects of psychoanalysis, whereas the Catholic press emphasized its application and its therapeutic potential. The Catholic press was also more likely to consider the potential of psychoanalysis to understand the psychic organization of the human personality. Moscovici noted that this sympathetic orientation reflected the historical period for Catholics, which was 'one in which psychoanalytic conceptions were being adapted to their own conceptions, making numerous articles, both critical and apologetic, necessary' (Moscovici, [1976] 2008, p. 211). Conversely, the Communist press was less sympathetic because its interpretation of reality was considered 'external to the way in which they interpret the real' (p. 211). Moscovici also noted the authors of the articles and remarked that those who had a strong religious or political stance tended to be less sympathetic. He quoted one article from *L'Humanité,* which had a more Communist orientation, describing psychoanalysis as 'a vile propaganda weapon' and stating that its analysts were 'trying to stupefy people with complexes' (p. 210). This detailed analysis of the press allowed Moscovici 'to get a clearer picture of how the press views psychoanalysis, to situate ideological groups with respect to it, and, finally, to trace the simple but basic outline of the social models that take it as a starting point' (pp. 213–214). Overall, the study revealed the value of employing different methods in studying social representations of psychoanalysis.

Health and illness: The next most important study was conducted by Claudine Herzlich (born 1932), who had worked as a research assistant on Moscovici's study and who emphasized the importance of the interview. Her study of social representations of health and illness (Herzlich, 1973) was conducted in the early 1960s, a period of rising social expectations and economic growth in France. Infant mortality was falling rapidly, and life expectancy was increasing. It was also a period of rapid urbanization and immigration from the former colonies. With the growth of the consumer society, there was sustained debate about health and quality of life (Bousquet & Pessin, 2003).

Herzlich's study was based on interviews conducted using a guide she described as being 'developed in terms of themes to be explored rather than in terms of closely formulated questions to be asked in a particular order' (p. 15). The interview transcripts were then analysed using a form of content analysis. This was guided by two approaches: first, by coding the interviews into themes and examining the relationships between themes; second, by considering cases, which were often complete interviews.

In his preface to the published work, Moscovici noted that there were 'no questionnaires, scales or statistical tests' (p. xiii). He continued that other studies may use 'more sophisticated methods and may be, in a technical sense, more professionally *respectable,* but they have been less well adapted to the object of their inquiry and therefore make a less genuine contribution to the process of science' (p. xiii–xiv). Moscovici was appealing to the wider psychological community in France, where more 'respectable' experimental methods had grown in strength (Santiago-Delefosse & del Rio Carral, 2017). Admittedly, in the French edition of her work, Herzlich (1969) did present a series of tables summarizing her main findings, although she did not conduct any statistical analyses.

Besides using the interview, an important aspect of Herzlich's work was the case-by-case analysis of the interview transcripts. This enabled her to develop an understanding of how the various themes were interconnected. She also included, in an appendix, a selection of extensive extracts from these interviews to illustrate these interconnections.

Herzlich was very cautious about the acceptability of her work. She concluded her introduction:

> As a matter of fact, with social psychology at its present stage, lacking any fully rigorous and satisfactory method of observation, strict methodological unity seems neither possible nor desirable. Indeed, it is through different methods of approach that the technique of investigation may be expected to advance. Such different methods of approach have, after all, but a single end – to make us think about the social image of health and illness and try to understand it (p. 16).

Her use of interviews was distinctive not just for its semi-structured design but also for the use of repeat interviews with a sub-sample and the application of a case method in her analysis. The case study is an important aspect of psychoanalysis, which was very prominent in French society at that time. Herzlich did not attempt a psychoanalytic interpretation of the cases but moved beyond what she described as a content analysis by exploring potential interconnections between themes within the various cases.

Mental illness: The third classic study was conducted by Denise Jodelet (born 1936), who carried out a detailed investigation of the social representations of mental illness in a rural community in France in the early 1970s (Jodelet, 1991). Mental healthcare had been reorganized in France in 1962, with a focus on prevention and treatment within the community (Verdoux & Tignol, 2003). This study is unique in that it combined a range of different methods in a case study of a particular community. In view of the extensive nature of this study, it is not surprising that it took four years to complete. Jodelet argued that it overcame the inadequacies of standard questionnaire and interview studies, which she listed:

> Notably the imposition on the population of the researcher's appreciation of the problems, his preconceptions and categories; the hypothesis of the transparency of speech but off from its productive context and its relationship to practice; the prevalence of accommodating or socially desirable replies or, again, rationalizations of the effectively adopted positions; the intuitive character of interpretations; hermeneutic interpretation of meaning without a mastery of the mechanisms which allow significations to emerge (p. 17).

These criticisms pre-empted much subsequent debate within qualitative research. She detailed, as well, the extensive nature of her interviews, which were guided by anthropological methods. She noted that in some of her interviews, she went 'from the particular to the general, via descriptions of patients and stories of everyday life, in order to obtain reflections on everyday illness' (p. 20). In this way, she aimed to discover 'secretly held ideas' which may have 'remained hidden in spontaneous discussion' (p. 21).

It is noteworthy that each of these classic studies was published as a monograph. This was a reflection of the intensive and extensive character of the research conducted. This character is one of the key features of social representation research, which has limited its appearance as popular journal articles. It is also a problem faced by social representation researchers, who are restricted by both funding and publication restraints. Researchers often compromise by publishing partial results, but this can limit a full understanding of the social representation of a particular phenomenon. This text does attempt to extract the key findings from a series of more extensive studies. It does however, deliberately detail the social context within which these studies were conducted.

3.5 Researching Social Representations

3.5.1 Collecting Data

Methodological principles: Moscovici (1984b, pp. 52–59) identified four methodological principles for conducting research on social representations. These are:

1. Material should be obtained from conversations normally exchanged in society. This can take various forms, from the open-ended interview to the focus group to the more free-flowing conversation obtained in various settings. This material can be supplemented by observations and other information about the participants' everyday lives.
2. Social representations should be considered a means of re-creating reality. The socially dynamic character is the central core of social representations. They are not fixed but rather reflect the active process of re-creating reality. In this sense, they are social constructions.
3. The character of social representations is especially revealed at times of crisis or change in society. When something disturbs our everyday life, that is the time to explore how people begin to make sense of their world. Certain phenomena (e.g., health and illness) are in a process of constant change.
4. People elaborating on social representations can be considered 'amateur scholars'. They bring together various sources of information and try to integrate them.

These basic principles provide a guide for particular approaches adopted in social representation research. Although both quantitative and qualitative methods have been used to investigate social representations, it is sufficient to briefly highlight certain aspects of qualitative research.

Participants: Research on social representations generally focuses on exploring the representations held by people in the wider community. This means moving out of the classic university setting and considering the diversity of representations in the community. When there is some evidence that social representations vary across certain sub-groups, the researcher will attempt to access information from those sub-groups. It is possible to replicate this search for diversity to a limited extent in university settings, which have increasingly diverse student populations. At all times, it is important to consider not only the details of the participants but also the socio-cultural setting within which the research takes place.

Interviews: Interviews remain the most common method within qualitative research. However, there has been ongoing refinement of this method (Flick, 2000b). An important issue in the conduct of interviews is the power dynamic between the interviewer and the interviewee. Zadeh (2017) has taken up this issue in her discussion of the importance of considering the dialogical nature of the interview. Previously, we described the dialogical triad, which forms the basis of understanding the development of social representations. This triad operates in the interview setting to the extent that the research participant (Alter) is replying to a question from the researcher (Ego) about some issue (Object).

It is for these reasons that the interview encounter is not presented as a neutral space but rather as an active social arena. Farr (1982) distinguished between the interview as a passive process and the interview as an active process. The researcher needs to be aware of this context and be prepared to offer conflicting perspectives. In analysing the interviews, the researcher is aware of the 'stance' adopted by the participant. On the one hand, the participants may strive to provide socially acceptable knowledge or, alternatively, attempt to convince the researcher of his/her stance.

One primary concern of the social representation researcher is to reduce the power differential between the researcher and the participant. This can be promoted in various ways. The researcher can deliberately take time to get to know the participant and engage with them in a conversational manner, possibly in a go-along interview, which can take different forms, including the walk-along and the ride-along (Kusenbach, 2003). The participant brings to the interview various experiences and apprehensions about the encounter. While demonstrating that they welcome different perspectives, some participants may feel intimidated by the setting. It is for this reason that repeat interviews or group discussions can be adopted.

Jovchelovitch (2007) suggests adopting a 'psychosocial' perspective in which the researcher approaches the interview encounter aware of these issues and is prepared to both listen to the participant and share their own perspective in a non-threatening manner. The alternative is to challenge the participants to provoke alternative perspectives. However, this may, in turn, silence the participants or have a longer-term negative impact. The aim of *conscienta* is to encourage the participants to see alternative perspectives. This approach is often seen as the core of adult education. It is also the core of political and therapeutic interventions.

Focus groups: Another development in interviews has been the use of focus groups. This approach is aimed at capturing how social representations develop in social interaction and explores the nature of arguments and disagreements within social representations. This approach attempts to break down the power imbalance between the researcher and the participants and instead promotes a more shared conversation within the group (Caillaud et al., 2022). Pictures and photographs can be used to encourage discussion in focus groups. The World Café approach is another recent development that can be used to foster discussion (Brown et al., 2007).

Ethnography: One problem with the use of interviews and other verbal methods of research is that it relies upon the ability of the participants to verbalize their representations. Further, it tends to present representations almost as rational constructions, devoid of emotional content. It is for this reason that researchers have attempted to integrate other forms of research.

Traditionally, ethnography as a method was used to investigate the social organization of communities, with the ethnographer's interpretive categories emerging through their reflexive analysis of observational data collected during fieldwork. Moscovici's definition of social representations as 'system(s) of values, ideas and practices' (p. xiii) encouraged a consideration of specific practices evident in a community, in the same way Herodotus had considered the importance of a community's social customs.

Media and art: While Moscovici, in his early work, considered the role of newspapers, in contemporary society, this has been largely superseded by social media, which is extensive and ever-present. Social representation theory is concerned with how the media, in its various forms, is structured and how different communities engage with it (see Cohen et al., 2022).

It can also consider how phenomena are represented in documents and in literary and artistic forms (e.g., Kaptein et al., 2020). Furthermore, we can consider historical and artistic images of certain phenomena and how these are connected with contemporary social representations.

Visual methods: A variety of visual methods have been used to explore social representations. These include drawings, photographs, and films. Drawing is a specific visual method that places the focus on the research participants, who are invited to draw a picture of a particular phenomenon, such as health or illness. It is a method that has been used in a number of studies on social representations.

In terms of social representations theory, Martikainen and Hakokönggäs (2022) described the process of drawing in terms of objectification. Drawing provides the research participant with the opportunity to objectify something that is more tenuous in form. Furthermore, drawing is an embodied process and, for that reason, may provide 'an insight into the multisensory, multimodal layers of knowledge and experience we are immersed in in our everyday lives but which are challenging to observe using "traditional" methods like interviews' (p. 11).

Participatory research: Much qualitative research has ignored the issue of power within the interview relationship and the extent to which this encourages or discourages the articulation of certain representations. Participatory research attempts to address this challenge by encouraging the researcher to be more collaborative in the research process. This can also include involving the subjects of the research more actively in the research process, such that they have the opportunity to shape the agenda and benefit from the research. This active engagement of participants in the research process provides them with an opportunity to reflect upon particular social representations (Campbell & Jovchelovitch, 2000; Cornish et al., 2014).

Participatory forms of drawing research include the involvement of the research participants in the analysis of the drawings. This can range from asking the participants to write about their drawings or talk about them. It provides an opportunity for the participants to reflect upon their ideas and practices (Martikainen & Hakokönggäs, 2022). The less formalized approach is particularly appropriate. For example, in her work on children's understanding of ethnicity, Howarth (2007) suggested that engaging children in conversation about their drawings was the most effective means of exploring their social representations.

3.5.2 Analysing Data

All data is subject to interpretation. Thus, the social representation researcher often adopts a combination of inductive and deductive approaches, coupled with attention to comparable research (Reichertz, 2014). Various strategies have been developed to strengthen the research.

Context: Social representations develop within certain times and places. It is thus necessary to consider the social and historical context within which social representations are being explored. For example, Moscovici's original study of social representations of psychoanalysis was conducted in France in the 1950s, when it was experiencing a growing interest. Lagache suggested that if the study had been conducted in the 1920s, the findings would have been somewhat different. Moscovici also noted that he had considered exploring social representations of Marxism, which was prominent in French society after the war. However, when he attempted to conduct such a study in the 1990s, he found little evidence that Marxism was of much interest to French people. The socio-political climate had changed (see Marková, 2023, p. 240). In their analyses, social representation researchers have been keen to grasp not just their understanding of the phenomenon but also the participants' location in society.

Thematic analysis: In analysing qualitative interviews in social representation research, the dominant approach has been the use of thematic analysis (Joffe, 2012). This analysis can have both an inductive and a deductive approach. The former approach follows careful coding of the interview transcripts, although excessive focus on correct coding can lead to a certain fetishism (Provencher, 2011). The latter approach emphasizes the importance of a theoretical perspective. Integrating these two approaches is the challenge. From an inductive perspective, the danger is moving too far from the data. From a deductive perspective, there is the need to mesh the data with the theoretical perspective. Further, there is the tension between description and interpretation. In early versions of qualitative research, the search was to reveal the voice of the research participants, particularly of those who had previously been ignored. It was argued that the researcher should adopt a disinterested stance in both data collection and analysis. However, all aspects of research take place within a social context, unlike the supposed 'social vacuum' that Tajfel (1972) condemned.

The important issue regarding the use of qualitative methods is the connection with theory. As Flick et al. (2015) emphasized: 'Data as well as statistical or other forms of results cannot per se be equated with a social representation'. There is a need for a 'theoretical inference and thus an interpretation which the researchers have to draw' (p. 79).

Discursive and rhetorical analysis: This approach focuses on the character of the interactive language used in conveying social representations. It is designed to identify the various discursive and rhetorical strategies used in specific contexts. Research participants engage in discussion with the Alter/Other, and this may give rise to various accounts. It is for this reason that the researcher needs to consider the context of data collection. As Zadeh (2017) argued: 'Rather than looking for consensus in participants' narratives, or producing reports that read like monologues, social representation researchers may do well to rather scrutinise the complexities and nuances in participants' accounts' (p. 267). Further, since participants may be reluctant to express certain perspectives within a specific context, the researcher needs to consider how to promote extensive contributions from the participants as well as a critical reading of the interview transcripts.

Narrative analysis: This approach is concerned with how the accounts provided by participants in a study have a particular narrative structure or tone, and how narratives are involved in the construction of social representations. One important criticism of Herzlich's work was that in her analysis, she ignored the narrative content of her participant's comments (László, 1997). However, the narrative structure of the interview material is apparent from reviewing the extracts that she reported. Another way of developing the narrative approach is to consider different levels of analysis (Murray, 2000). Thus, you can consider the use of narrative in social interaction and in the organization of social representations.

Hidden representations: While the focus of research is on what the person says and does, the researcher is also alert to more hidden dimensions. Furthermore, how the persons express their views may conceal their social representations, which may be 'buried under the layers of words and images floating in people's minds' (Moscovici, 1994, p. 168).

A way of conceptualizing this silence is the idea of a 'mute zone' in social representations. This approach was developed by Deschamps and Guimelli (2002), with the suggestion that certain elements in a social representation are masked and thus made mute, not expressed in certain situations. In their review of this concept, Rateau and Monaco (2021) noted that Moscovici (1961) had observed this process in his original study, with some people not mentioning certain elements of psychoanalysis, especially the libido concept, which Moscovici suggested was due to broader values concerning sexuality. This would suggest that the researcher needs to explore what concepts are not disclosed in interviews. In the same way, Jacques Rancière, in his essay *Figures of History*, described the duty of the artist as being to show 'what can't be seen, what lies beneath the visible' (Stepanova, 2021, p. 50).

Triangulation: With the preference for multiple methods, social representation researchers could be accused of ignoring epistemological and theoretical differences. An approach to reconciling such differences has been the use of the concept of triangulation. The term was originally used in military and marine contexts to describe how to situate an object using two or more points (Wagner et al., 1999). It was then introduced into the social sciences by Denzin (1970) in the debate about validity in qualitative research.

However, within social representation theory, there is greater acceptance of different social realities. Flick (1992) has argued that triangulation goes beyond searching for a single truth; rather, it aims at 'combining several perspectives in a systematic way' (p. 77). Thus, it takes into consideration the different methodological, epistemological, and theoretical assumptions underlying the various perspectives and aims to develop a more sophisticated understanding of the phenomenon. It is this concern with integrating different methods that has led social representation theorists to value the importance of triangulation (Flick, 2017). Furthermore, Flick (1992) has argued that the full potential of triangulation is reached when different methods embody different theoretical perspectives. He subsequently termed this approach 'systematic triangulation' to highlight that it considers the different assumptions of the various perspectives rather than the simple accumulation of methods (Flick, 2017).

An overview of the different approaches to triangulation has been developed by Sabine Caillaud et al. (2019), which is summarized in Table 3.1. This contrasts three approaches to triangulation: methodological—as a strategy of validation; interdisciplinary—where different approaches are combined; and systematic—which takes into consideration the theoretical and epistemological differences in the methods. A systematic approach opens up the critical potential of social representation theory. By highlighting the different social representations, it can question the dominance of particular representations and how certain groups may support these, despite their adverse consequences. An important feature of systematic

Table 3.1 Different triangulation approaches

Types	*Strategy of validation*	*Pragmatic*	*Systematic*
What is it?	Criteria of validity	Step to more knowledge	Extension of research programme
How is it planned?	Combining qualitative and quantitative	Pragmatic combination	Systematic selection and linking to theory
How are results considered?	Convergence as validity criteria	Discrepancies & contradictions included	Source of extra knowledge

Source Caillaud et al. (2019).

triangulation is the awareness that different representations can be simultaneously present, as in cognitive polyphasia.

Reflexivity: More recently, within qualitative research, there has been debate about the role of the researcher in conducting and analysing interviews. There has been an appeal for greater reflexivity, such that the researcher considers the role they play. While this is an important consideration, social representation researchers have attempted to address this by often adopting different qualitative and quantitative methods. For example, they can combine interviews with focus groups and media analysis. The researcher needs to consider how they are embedded in a network of representations and how these influence their interpretations (Flick et al., 2015). They can also adopt a more participatory form of research, such that the research participants have the opportunity to challenge certain interpretations of the data. Critical reflexivity involves going beyond the immediate research agenda and, through debate and dialogue with participants, opening up alternative representations and ways of social transformation (Guareschi & Jovchelovitch, 2004).

3.6 Orientation

This chapter reviewed the main theoretical tenets of social representation theory, its developments, and the ways it has been used to investigate it. It is apparent that, although the basic tenets of social representation theory have remained consistent, it has resulted in a very fruitful expansion of our understanding of the processes underlying them. The innovative initial research projects need to be considered within their socio-historical context. Certain other theoretical approaches have also been considered for their potential linkages with social representation theory.

The research methods used have expanded from a reliance on interview methods to a more expansive use of quantitative and qualitative methods. The expansion of theoretical and methodological connections is not evidence of a weakening of conceptual coherence but rather an acceptance of the complexity of our social understandings. These interconnections are developed in the concept of triangulation (Flick, 1992; Caillaud et al., 2019).

This review has provided an orientation to the various research studies considered in subsequent chapters. In these studies, different theoretical approaches and methods have been used to explore social representations of health and illness among people of different ages and in different socio-historic contexts. In particular, a more historical and socio-cultural approach is adopted to explore the connections between the context and the social representations of health and illness. We consider the importance of the historical period within which the research was conducted. This includes consideration of such cultural forms as music and literature. Rather than searching for constancy in how we develop social representations of health and illness, we will consider how these change over time. In some ways, this is similar to the approach suggested by Wundt in the development of his *Völkerspsychologie*.

References

Abric, J.-C. (2001). A structural approach to social representations. In K. Deaux & G. Philogène (Eds.), *Representations of the social* (pp. 42–47). Blackwell.

Apfelbaum, E. (2009). Against the tide: Making waves and breaking silences. In L. P. Mos (Ed.), *History of psychology in autobiography* (pp. 1–36). Springer.

Augoustinos, M. (2001). Social categorization: Towards theoretical integration. In K. Deaux & G. Philogène (Eds.), *Representations of the social* (pp. 201–216). Blackwell.

Batel, S., & Castro, P. (2018). Reopening the dialogue between the theory of social representations and discursive psychology for examining the construction and transformation of meaning in discourse and communication. *British Journal of Social Psychology*, *57*(4), 732–753.

Batel, S., & Castro, P. (2019). Still a matter of dialogue: A response to Potter's, Augoustinos's, and Jovchelovitch's commentaries. *British Journal of Social Psychology, 58*(2), 428–434.

Baubion-Broye, A., Lapeyre, M., & Malrieu, P. (1977). Remarques sur la notion de représentation sociale. *Psychologie Et Education, 3*, 37–56.

Bauer, M. W., & Gaskell, G. (1999). Towards a paradigm for research on social representations. *Journal for the Theory of Social Behaviour, 29*(2), 163–186.

Bhugra, D., Smith, A., Liebrenz, M., Ventriglio, A., Gnanapragasam, S. M., Buadze, A., Pemberton, M., & Poulter, D. (2023). "Otherness", otherism, discrimination, and health inequalities: Entrenched challenges for modern psychiatric disciplines. *International Review of Psychiatry, 35*(3–4), 234–241.

Bousquet, G., & Pessin, A. (2003). Culture and identity in post-war France. In N. Hewitt (Ed.), *The Cambridge companion to modern French culture* (pp. 41–60). Cambridge University Press.

Brown, J., Homans, K., & Isaacs, D. (2007). The world café. In D. Holman, T. Devane, & S. Cady (Eds.), *The change handbook* (2nd ed., pp. 179–194). Berrett-Koehler.

Caillaud, S., Doumergue, M., Preau, M., Haas, V., & Kalampalikis, N. (2019). The past and present of triangulation and social representations theory: A crossed history. *Qualitative Research in Psychology, 16*(3), 375–391.

Caillaud, S., Ginguene, S., Maharjan, S. M., Koirala, G., Tonon, B., & Le Roch, K. (2024). Social representations of the undernourished child and health-seeking behaviour in Nepal: From othering to different types of otherness. *Journal of Community & Applied Social Psychology, 32*(2), 273–287.

Caillaud, S., Kalampalikis, N., & Doumergue, M. (2022). Designing focus groups. In U. Flick (Ed.), *The SAGE handbook of qualitative research design* (pp. 684–699). Sage.

Campbell, C., & Jovchelovich, S. (2000). Health, community and development: Towards a social psychology of participation. *Journal of Community and Applied Social Psychology, 10*(4), 255–270.

Cohen, G., Bessin, M., & Gaymard, S. (2022). Social representations, media and iconography: A semidiscursive analysis of Facebook posts related to the COVID-19 pandemic. *European Journal of Communication, 37*(6), 629–645.

Cornish, F., Gillespie, A., & Zittoun, T. (2014). Collaborative analysis of qualitative Data. In U. Flick (Ed.), *The SAGE handbook of qualitative data analysis* (pp. 79–93). Sage.

de Rosa, A. S. (1987). The social representations of mental illness in children and adults. In W. Doise & S. Mocovici (Eds.), *Current issues in European social psychology* (Vol. 2, pp. 47–138). Cambridge University Press.

de Saint-Laurent, C. (2018). Thinking through time: From collective memories to collective futures. In C. de Saint-Laurent, S. Obradovic, & K. R. Carriere (Eds.), *Imagining collective futures* (pp. 59–81). Palgrave.

Denzin, N. (1970). *The research act: A theoretical introduction to sociological methods*. McGraw-Hill.
Deschamps, J. C., & Guimelli, C. (2002). La composante émotionelle des représentations sociales: émotions rapportées et tendances à l'action dans une étude comparative des représentations sociales de l'insécurité en France et en Suisse. *Nouvelle Revue de Psychologie Sociale*, *1*(1), 78–84.
Doise, W. (1986). *Levels of explanation in social psychology*. Cambridge University Press.
Doise, W., & Mugny, G. (1975). Recherche sociogénétiques sur la co-ordination d'actions independantes. *Revue Suisse de Psychologie*, *34*, 160–174.
Doise, W., Clemence, A., & Lorenzi-Cioldi, F. (1993). *The quantitative analysis of social representations*. Hemel Hempstead, Harvester Wheatsheaf.
Duveen, G. (2001a). Representations, identities and resistance. In K. Deaux & G. Philogène (Eds.), *Representations of the social*. Blackwell.
Duveen, G. (2001b). Genesis and structure: Piaget and Moscovici. In F. Buschini & N. Kalampalikis (Eds.), *Penser la Vie, le Social, la Nature* (pp. 163–174). Éditions de la Maison des sciences de l'homme.
Duveen, G. (2007). Culture and social representations. In J. Valsiner & A. Rosa (Eds.), *The Cambridge handbook of sociocultural psychology* (pp. 543–559). Cambridge University Press.
Edwards, D., & Potter, J. (1992). *Discursive psychology*. Sage.
Erpenbeck, J. (2023). *Kairos*. Granta.
Farr, R. M. (1982). Interviewing: The social psychology of the inter-view. In F. Fransella (Ed.), *Psychology and people: A tutorial text. Psychology for professional groups*. Palgrave.
Fishbein, M., & Ajzen, I. (1975). *Belief, attitude, intention and behavior: An introduction to theory and research*. Addison-Wesley.
Flick, U. (1992). Triangulation revisited: Strategy of validation or alternative? *Journal for the Theory of Social Behaviour*, *22*(2), 175–192.
Flick, U. (2000a). Episodic interviewing. In M. W. Bauer & G. Gaskell (Eds.), *Qualitative researching with text, image and sound* (pp. 75–92). Sage.
Flick, U. (2000b). Qualitative inquiries into social representations of health. *Journal of Health Psychology*, *5*(3), 315–324.
Flick, U. (2017). Triangulation. In N. Denzin & Y. Lincoln (Eds.), *The SAGE handbook of qualitative research* (pp. 443–461). Sage.
Flick, U., Foster, J., & Caillaud, S. (2015). Researching social representations. In G. Sammut, E. Andreouli, G. Gaskell, & J. Valsiner (Eds.), *The Cambridge handbook of social representations* (pp. 64–82). Cambridge University Press.
Foucault, M. (1961 [1965]). *Madness and Civilization [Folie Et Déraison: Histoire de la Folie À L'âge Classique]*. Pantheon.

Foucault, M. (2020). *Power: The essential works of Michel Foucault 1954–1984.* Penguin.
Gough, B., McFadden, M., & McDonald, M. (2013). *Critical social psychology.* An introduction (2nd edn.). Palgrave.
Guareschi, P. A., & Jovchelovitch, S. (2004). Participation, health and the development of community resources in Southern Brazil. *Journal of Health Psychology, 9*(2), 311–322.
Hall, S. (1997). *Representation: Cultural representations and signifying practices.* Sage.
Heider, F. (1958). *The psychology of interpersonal relations.* John Wiley.
Herzlich, C. (1973). *Health and illness. A social psychological analysis.* London: Academic Press (Original: *Santé et Maladie: Analyse d'une Réprésentation Sociale.* Paris: Mouton, 1969).
Hewitt, N. (2003). Introduction: French culture and society in the twentieth century. In N. Hewitt (Ed.), *The Cambridge companion to modern French culture* (pp. 1–16). Cambridge University Press.
Holton, G. (1978). *The scientific imagination: Case studies.* Cambridge University Press.
Howarth, C. (2006). A social representation is not a quiet thing: Exploring the critical potential of social representations theory. *British Journal of Social Psychology, 45*(1), 65–86.
Howarth, C. (2007). It's not their fault that they have that skin colour, is it?" Young British children and the possibilities for contesting racialized representations. In G. Moloney & I. Walker (Eds.), *Social representations and identity: Content, process, and power* (pp. 131–156). Palgrave Macmillan.
Howarth, C., Andreouli, E., & Kessi, S. (2014). Social representations and the politics of participation. In P. Nesbitt-Larking, C. Kinnvall, T. Capelos, & H. Dekker (Eds.), *The Palgrave handbook of global political psychology* (pp. 19–38). Palgrave.
Jodelet, D. (1991). *Madness and social representations. Living with the mad in one French community.* University of California Press.
Jodelet, D. (2012a). Interconnections between social representations and intervention. In A. de Rosa (Ed.), *Social representations in the 'Social Arena'* (pp. 77–88). Routledge.
Jodelet, D. (2012b). About the impact of the theory of social representations. In R. Permandelli, D. Jodelet, & T. Sugiman (Eds.), *Alternative production of knowledge and social representations.* University of Indonesia Press.
Joffe, H. (1996). The shock of the new: A psychodynamic extension of social representations theory. *Journal for the Theory of Social Behaviour, 26*(2), 197–219.
Joffe, H. (2012). Thematic analysis. In D. Harper & A. R. Thompson (Eds.), *Qualitative research in mental health and psychotherapy: A guide for students and practitioners* (pp. 209–223). Wiley-Blackwell.

Jovchelovitch, S. (2007). *Knowledge in context. Representations, community and culture*. Routledge.
Jovchelovitch, S., & Bauer, M. W. (2000). Narrative interviewing. In M. W. Bauer & G. Gaskell (Eds.), *Qualitative researching with text, image and sound* (pp. 57–74). Sage.
Kaptein, A. A., Meulenberg, F., & Murray, M. (2020). Artistic representations of infectious disease. *Psychology, Health and Medicine*, *25*(4), 492–496.
Kusenbach, M. (2003). Street phenomenology: The Go-along as ethnographic research tool. *Ethnography*, *4*, 455–485.
László, J. (1997). Narrative organization of social representations. *Papers on Social Representations*, *6*(2), 154–167.
Lenin, V. I. (1902). *What is to be done?* Progress.
Leventhal, H., Meyer, D., & Nerenz, D. (1980). The commonsense representations of illness changes. In S. Rachman (Ed.), *Contributions to medical psychology, Vol. 2*. Pergamon.
Lord, A. (1986). *Our dead behind us: Poems*. W.W. Norton.
Marková, I. (2003). *Dialogicality and social representations. The dynamics of mind*. Cambridge University Press.
Marková, I. (2023). *The making of a dialogical theory. Social representations and communication*. Cambridge University Press.
Martikainen, J., & Hakokönggäs, E. (2022). Drawing as a method of researching social representations. *Qualitative Research*, *23*(4), 981–999.
Maxwell, J. A., & Chmiel, M. (2014). Generalization in and from qualitative analysis. In U. Flick (Ed.), *The SAGE handbook of qualitative data analysis* (pp. 540–553). Sage.
Midlands Psychology Group. (2022). *Outsight: Psychology, politics and social justice*. PCCS Books.
Moscovici, S., & Vignaux, G. (1994/2000). The concept of themata. In S. Moscovici, *Social representations* (edited and trans. by G. Duveen) (pp. 156–183). London: Polity.
Moscovici, S. (1993). *The invention of society*. Polity.
Moscovici, S. (2008, [1976]). Psychoanalysis: Its Image and Its Public. *[English Translation of La Psychoanalyse, Son Image Et Son Image, 1976]*. Polity Press.
Moscovici, S. (1961). *La Psychanalyse: Son Image Et Son Public*. Presses Universitaires de France.
Moscovici, S. (1984a). The myth of the lonely paradigm: A rejoinder. *Social Research*, *51*(4), 939–967.
Moscovici, S. (1984b). The phenomenon of social representations. In R. M. Farr & S. Moscovici (Eds.), *Social representations* (pp. 3–70). Cambridge University Press.
Moscovici, S. (1985). *The Age of the Crowd. A Historical Treatise on Mass Psychology*. Cambridge University Press.

Moscovici, S. (1988). Notes towards a description of social representations. *European Journal of Social Psychology, 18*(3), 211–250.
Moscovici, S. (1994). Social representations and pragmatic communication. *Social Science Information, 33*(2), 163–177.
Moscovici, S. (1998a). The history and actuality of social representations. In U. Flick (Ed.), *The psychology of the social* (pp. 209–247). Cambridge University Press.
Moscovici, S. (1998b). Social consciousness and its history. *Culture & Psychology, 4*(3), 411–429.
Moscovici, S. (2000). In G. Duveen (Ed.), *Social representations. Explorations in social psychology.* Polity.
Moscovici, S. (2002). Pensée stigmatique et pensée symbolique: Deux formes élémentaires de la pensée sociale. In C. Garnier (Ed.), *Les Formes de la Pensée Sociale.* Presses Universitaires de France.
Moscovici, S., & Marková, I. (1998). Presenting social representations: A conversation. *Culture & Psychology, 4*(3), 371–410.
Moscovici, S., & Marková, I. (2000). Ideas and their development: A dialogue between Serge Moscovici and Ivana Marková. In S. Moscovici & G. Duveen (Eds.), *Social pepresentations: Explorations in social psychology* (pp. 208–223). Polity Press.
Murray, M., & McMillan, C. (1993). Gender differences in perceptions of cancer. *Journal of Cancer Education, 8*(1), 53–62.
Murray, M. (1993). Social and cognitive representations of health and illness. In H. Schroder, K. Reschke, M. Johnson, & S. Maes (Eds.), *Health psychology—potential in diversity* (pp. 124–131).
Murray, M. (1997). A narrative approach to health psychology: Background and potential. *Journal of Health Psychology, 2*(1), 9–20.
Murray, M. (2000). Levels of narrative analysis in health psychology. *Journal of Health Psychology, 5*(3), 331–342.
Murray, M. (2002). Connecting narrative and social representation theory in health research. *Social Science Information, 41*(4), 653–673.
Murray, M. (2024). Narrative psychology. In J. A. Smith (Ed.), *Qualitative psychology: A practical guide to research methods* (4th edn., pp. 85–107). Sage.
Piaget, J. (1932). *The moral judgment of the child.* Harcourt, Brace.
Potter, J., & Wetherell, M. (1987). *Discourse and social psychology. Beyond attitudes and behaviour.* Sage.
Provencher, C. (2011). Towards a better understanding of cognitive polyphasia. *Journal for the Theory of Social Behaviour, 41*(4), 377–395.
Rateau, P., & Lo Monaco, G. (2021). The mute zone of social representations and the effects of (un)masking: Review and prospects. *RUDN Journal of Psychology and Pedagogics, 18*(2), 375–390.

Reichertz, J. (2014). Induction, deduction, abduction. In U. Flick (Ed.), *The SAGE handbook of qualitative data analysis* (pp. 123–135). Sage.

Sarbin, T. R. (Ed.). (1986). *Narrative psychology. The storied nature of human conduct.* Praeger.

Selbin, E. (2010). *Revolution, rebellion, resistance: The power of story.* Zed Books.

Tajfel, H. (1972). Experiments in a vacuum. In J. Israel & H. Tajfel (Eds.), *The context of social psychology. A critical assessment* (pp. 69–119). Academic Press.

Tajfel, H. (1978). Social categorization, social identity and social comparison. In H. Tajfel (Ed.), *Differentiation between social groups* (pp. 61–76). Academic Press.

Tajfel, H., & Turner, J. C. (1986). The social identity theory of intergroup behaviour. In S. Worchel & W. G. Austin (Eds.), *The psychology of intergroup relations* (pp. 7–24). Nelson-Hall.

Taylor, C. (2016). *The language animal: The full shape of the human linguistic capacity.* Harvard University Press.

Verdoux, H., & Tignol, J. (2003). Focus on psychiatry in France. *British Journal of Psychiatry, 183*(5), 466–471.

Vidal-Niquet, P. (2001). Deux notes sur l'oeuvre de Serge Moscovici. In F. Buschini & N. Kalampalikis (Eds.), *Penser la Vie, Le Social, La Nature.* Éditions de la Maison des Sciences de l'Homme.

Wagner, W., Duveen, G., Farr, R., Jovchelovitch, S., Lorenzi-Cioldi, F., Marková, I., & Rose, D. (1999). Theory and method of social representations. *Asian Journal of Social Psychology, 2*, 95–125.

Wagoner, B. (2015). Collective remembering as a process of social representation. In G. Sammut, E. Andreouli, G. Gaskell, & J. Valsiner (Eds.), *The Cambridge handbook of social representations* (pp. 143–162). Cambridge University Press.

Whyte, J. (2018). "A new geography of defence": The birth of psychological warfare. *Political Geography, 67*, 32–45.

Winskell, K. (2021). Social representations theory and young Africans' creative narratives about HIV/AIDS, 1997–2014. *Journal for the Theory of Social Behaviour, 51*(1), 164–182.

PART II

Health and Illness

CHAPTER 4

Health and Illness Among Young People

Childhood and adolescence are periods of rapid social and psychological development. During this time, we become aware of ourselves and our relationships with others. This chapter begins by considering different approaches to the study of child development. It then focuses on the social representations of health and illness among children and young people and how these connect with their families and broader socio-cultural milieu. It highlights the importance of the setting within which the research is conducted and the research methods adopted.

4.1 Youth

In the modern world, youth is generally considered the period in human development from childhood through adolescence to early adulthood. Research interest in this period really grew in the 1960s, a time that marked the growth of modern youth culture in Western society. This was the time when the post-war economy in the Western world was experiencing sustained economic growth, with rising living standards, the expansion of healthcare and education provision and greater opportunities for young people.

A major initiative in explaining children's understanding of the world was the work of Piaget (1932). He posited that human cognitive development moves through a series of stages. The first of these, which occurs

M. Murray, *Social Representations, Health and Illness*,
https://doi.org/10.1007/978-3-031-98494-5_4

in the first two years of life, is the sensorimotor stage, in which children learn to know the world through movement and sensations. This is followed by the pre-operational stage (2–7 years), in which children learn to think symbolically, using drawings and words to represent the world. Then there is the concrete operational stage (7–11 years), in which children begin to think logically about concrete events. The formal operational stage (11+ years) is when children learn to think abstractly. While this theory was a major innovation, it made limited reference to social circumstances. Although he is often described as an 'interactionist' because of his idea that children develop cognitively through acting on the world, he did not consider the impact of the broader socio-cultural environment on the child (Birns, 1972). Conversely, Henri Wallon (1879–1962), a contemporary French child researcher, while accepting the idea of stages in child development emphasized the importance of the social environment and the child's use of language (van der Veer, 1996).

The importance of the social environment was taken up by some American child psychologists, although they continued to emphasize the idea of stages in human development. Erik Erikson prefigured this movement with the publication, in 1950, of *Childhood and Society*. Working from a psychoanalytic perspective, he argued that we proceed through eight stages of development characterized by ongoing conflict between biological and sociocultural forces. Within each of the youth stages (infancy, toddlerhood, early and late childhood, adolescence and early adulthood), there is a psychosocial crisis, such as that between trust and mistrust in the infancy stage. If the individual successfully overcomes this crisis, they carry a certain virtue into the next stage. In the transition from infancy to toddlerhood, the virtue is hope. This theory very much reflected the North American cultural context and the widespread interest in psychoanalytic theory at that time.

Building upon these ideas, Levinson (1978) developed another stageist approach to social development, arguing that there are a series of stages in human life, moving from pre-adulthood, early adulthood, middle adulthood and late adulthood. Initially, Levinson's theory was based upon interviews with men, but he subsequently supplemented it with interviews with women, who he argued were more concerned with domestic rather than work issues. However, there remained the problem that his work was based on a limited sample of middle-aged North Americans in the 1970s. While these approaches were an important contribution to our understanding of children's thinking and young people's social development, a major concern is their assumption that they move through a fixed series of stages. The alternative is to see children as being born into a social world and developing an understanding of that world through interaction with others.

This is something that social representation theory addresses. It argues that children are born into a world that is bounded by social representations of their world and their place in it. As they develop, they learn about these social representations and internalize them as features of their social identity. As Duveen (2001a) said:

> Even before they are born, at times even before they are conceived, children are already the objects of the hopes, fears, aspirations, and anxieties of the people who will become their parents ... A child is always a construction before it is a reality, but a construction of others, and through this construction its parents and others extend to it a social identity, they locate it in a social space (p. 259).

In their study of children's development, Lloyd and Duveen (1992) used a combination of methods, including ethnography, interviews and standardized measures, to develop an understanding of the development of social representations of gender among primary school children. In play activities, there was a clear demarcation of masculine and feminine activities that were endowed with power qualities. Masculine activities and things were associated with greater power. However, there were disputes between the children over involvement in activities and access to resources, with girls challenging the traditional gender differences and teachers attempting to provide equal access to resources. Children may be born into certain social representations of gender, but upon entry to different institutions, such as schools, they begin to engage in challenges to these representations. Social representations of gender may impose a distinction upon the children, but it is one that is re-negotiated on an ongoing basis in social interaction. However, this was not easy to change, as the children tended to enforce the traditional gender differentiation themselves. This illustrated the difficulty we experience in challenging hegemonic social representations.

These social representations of gender become psychologically active through the social identities of the children. The children enact these social identities through their everyday social interactions and their physical activities. '[F]or young children meanings are more clearly established through their practical activity than through intellectual understanding' (Lloyd & Duveen, 1992, p. 179). This was part of the process of ontogenesis. However, it is important to recognize that this process is not universal but is socially and historically located.

A further indication of children's understanding of their social location was explored in a study by Jovchelovitch et al. (2013). They emphasized that much previous research had adopted an asocial Piagetian cognitivist perspective, which focused on universal stages of development rather than considering the socio-cultural context. As they stated: 'children's knowledge develops embedded and shaped by the psycho-social dynamics of self-other relations, modes of communication, and the cultural patterns of different public spheres' (p. 327). Thus, their understandings are not an inferior form of knowledge but one that is linked to their everyday social world.

Their study focused on how children from four different cultural contexts (Germany, Mexico, Brazil and Romania), of varying ages and social backgrounds, understood the concept of a public place. To assess their understanding, the researchers employed a mixed-method design that included ethnographic observation with field notes documenting the children's everyday activities, a drawing exercise in which the children were asked to create an image of their local place, and a subsequent short interview about their drawings. The drawings were categorized into three groups: subjective, intersubjective and objective. Statistical analysis of this categorization revealed differences in the children's understanding of place based on age, social class and cultural background.

Of particular importance, the more objective view of the public place was one associated with Western public spaces defined by affluence and individualism. This link with cultural context illustrates how 'children's knowledge is irreducible to an under-developed version of adult knowledge' (p. 340). Rather, they are connected with the children's experience of public places. It is not the typical Piagetian development from subjective to objective views of the public place but one that is socially immersed. This contrast between the cognitivist and the more social interactionist approaches to human development is reflected in studies of the development of understandings of health and illness.

4.2 Young Children in North America and Europe, 1980–2020

The earliest research on understanding children's representations of health and illness drew upon Piaget's approach to cognitive development. In a study conducted in the United States, Bibace and Walsh (1980) used this framework to explore the explanations of illness offered by children of different ages. The method adopted followed the 'clinical method' developed by Piaget to elicit causal reasoning in a sample of children. The children were individually interviewed and asked a series of questions about various illnesses and were asked to explain them. Analysis of the children's replies was organized into three main categories. The younger (4-year-olds) children's replies were categorized more as pre-logical, in that the children were unable to provide an explanation. The older children (7-year-olds) used more concrete-logical explanations, which emphasized contamination and internalization. The oldest (11-year-olds) children's replies were categorized as formal-operational explanations, which introduced physiological and psychophysiological processes. The authors concluded that this demonstrated that children's understanding of illness was linked to the Piagetian stage of cognitive development and, together, showed a shift from more subjective to more objective explanations. However, this approach considered children's understanding of health and illness in an abstract sense, with little reference to their experience.

Alternative approaches, which placed more emphasis on the experience of the children, were proposed. The British psychologist Christine Eiser (1989) considered two such 'functionalist' approaches proposed by two American developmental psychologists. The first was the script approach proposed by Nelson (1986), which argued that children develop a particular cognitive representation of events in their world. Scripts are representations of episodes containing a series of events—almost like narratives. Eiser et al. (1989) asked a group of five-year-olds and another group of eight-year-olds to describe a visit to the doctor. They found that even the younger children could give an account indicating their structured knowledge of the events. These scripts were more elaborated among the older children. Another approach is that of conceptual change proposed by Carey (1985). She interviewed children aged 4–10 years about their understanding of the human body and argued that while younger children talk about bodily systems in terms of wants and beliefs, older children had a theory of the body based upon its uses (e.g., you eat because it's dinner time). Thus, the child develops an understanding of the body based upon personal experience. However, these studies made limited reference to how the children's understandings developed in social interaction with others and the broader socio-cultural context.

An attempt to address this inadequacy was developed by two French Canadian psychologists, Sylvie Jutras and Jocelyn Bisson (1994). They adopted a social phenomenological approach, which was concerned with elucidating the character of the children's 'life world'. Jutras and Bisson described their approach as 'more pragmatic, less preoccupied by epistemology and issues of power and more oriented to the individual'[1] (p. 8, trans.) than social representation theory. They coupled their approach with an ecological orientation, taking into consideration the role of the family, the media and other societal influences. They also noted that earlier studies had asked children about health in the abstract, which children found difficult to grasp.

In their study, Jutras and Bisson conducted a large interview survey of over 500 children aged 5–12 years residing in Québec. They asked the children to think of a healthy person they knew and then to provide some details about why that person was healthy. They found that the majority of 5- to 6-year-olds were able to provide details about good health. Among children of all ages, the most common criteria for health were coded into four main categories: Functionality (sports, absence of illness, school work, etc.), well-being (energy, good mental health), lifestyle (good diet), bodily factors (reference to body, complexion) and a minor category of social relations. The use of energy, absence of illness, complexion and bodily manifestations increased with age. In this study, the children had an opportunity to connect health with their real-life experiences in their descriptions of another child they knew. This illustrated that children develop an understanding of health in context. They also noted some gender differences, with boys being more likely to refer to sporting activities in their definitions of health, while girls referred more frequently to mental health and good diet. Jutras and Bisson suggested that these gender differences reflected the different socialization experiences of boys and girls.

[1] 'plus pragmatiques, moins préoccupés par l'épistémologie et les rapports de pouvoir et plus orientés vers l'individu' (p. 8).

Another study in Québec by Sylvie Normandeau et al. (1998) further developed this phenomenological approach. A total of 1674 children aged 5–12 years from different socio-economic backgrounds and residing in either Montréal or Sherbrooke (a smaller city in Québec) and its rural hinterland participated in the study. These children were individually interviewed about their understanding of health in the context of their everyday lives. Specifically, they were asked to explore the health of their friends and what they could do in their everyday lives to promote health. The children's replies were subjected to content analysis, which contributed to the development of three main categories. The first was labelled functionality and included practicing sports and activities as well as the absence of illness. The second was mental health and included well-being (looking healthy, having energy and feeling good) and relationships. The third category was labelled lifestyle and included a healthy diet. This confirmed the importance of social and physical engagement in the children's understanding of health. In addition, the children's age and living arrangements were important, with older children emphasizing a healthy lifestyle, physical activities and mental health, while those from more middle-class homes placed more emphasis on a healthy lifestyle. They did not note any gender differences. From a social representation perspective, it would seem that the children anchored health in everyday physical activities and how these were performed in their local environment.

This study also explored evidence of mental health referents in the children's descriptions of health (Jutras et al., 1998). The researchers identified seven dimensions of mental health: social support, harmonious interpersonal relationships, expression of positive emotions, school involvement, high morale, relaxation and nonspecific mental health. Social support and harmonious interpersonal relationships were referred to most frequently, indicating the anchoring of mental health in social relationships and support.

Another study conducted in Québec examined conceptions of wellness in the families of children with diabetes (Jutras et al., 2003). The study consisted of structured interviews with 53 mothers, 53 children with diabetes and 55 siblings. These interviews asked questions about both diabetes and wellness. The responses were content analysed and certain differences between the three groups were identified. The mothers more frequently mentioned 'positive attitude' in their definitions of wellness, referring to joy in life, a sense of humour, good mood and optimism. Mothers also more frequently mentioned observable cues to well-being, such as a healthy-looking complexion and bright eyes. More than one-third of the mothers mentioned the capacity to express emotions and opinions, which was not mentioned by the children. The siblings more frequently mentioned performance within the social and family setting. Of particular note was the finding that the absence of tension or family conflict was mentioned more frequently by the children with diabetes. Together, this study emphasized how wellbeing is embedded within the family setting and the importance of harmonious relations.

Other studies have moved beyond reliance on interviews as the main method of data collection, and they have also given more consideration to the social lives of the children. A study in London contrasted three different approaches to obtaining insight into children's perceptions of health: write-only, draw-and-write and label-and-write (Pridmore & Bendelow, 1995). The study involved 126 9- to 10-year-old boys and girls from three schools, two of which were in the poorest borough of London and one in a neighbouring borough. The children were asked to describe what made a child healthy. The children identified a healthy diet, sport and hygiene as important for health. In representing the causes of illness, the children also mentioned poor diet, lack of exercise, lack of sleep, poor hygiene, smoking/alcohol/drug/substance abuse, not taking care and diseases. Smoking included cigarettes, 'spliffs' and 'ganga', while drugs included injecting heroin, sniffing glue/solvents, cocaine and taking ecstasy. The category 'not taking care' referred to accidents such as burning, violence, gangs, bullying and getting too hot, cold or wet. They found that the write-only task provided the most detail, but the draw-and-write task showed how concepts were related. The label-and-write task provided more details on the physical signs of health. They concluded that no single method was best, but a careful use of a combination of drawing and writing could balance the strengths and limitations of the different methods. The reference to negative social experiences and the use of drugs reflected the disadvantaged area in which the children lived.

In a Hungarian study (Piko & Bak, 2006), 126 primary school children aged 8–11 years, who were residents of a small town, were asked to draw or write about health and illness. Their replies were coded into two broad categories: biomedical and holistic, which were equally common. In addition, they also referred to a healthy lifestyle, such as exercise and diet. With regard to illness, the children frequently referred to the causes of illness, such as contagion and contamination. In terms of health promotion, it was noted that the children also emphasized equilibrium, harmony and a balance between themselves and their environment. They also noted the lack of reference to such social factors as violence and homelessness as causes of illness, reflecting the more tranquil character of the small town in which the children lived.

A study in Greece (Mouratidi et al., 2016) produced similar findings. In this study, a sample of 347 children aged 5–11 years and 220 adults from a medium-sized city were asked to draw images of health and illness and to give a title to their drawings. These drawings were classified into three categories: biomedical, psychosocial and lifestyle. The most common categories for illness were biomedical and psychosocial, with the biomedical category being especially common among the children. For health, the most common categories for children were psychosocial and lifestyle, whereas for adults, it was especially psychosocial. The younger children made less reference to lifestyle factors. The greater reference to biomedical in the children's drawings of illness would indicate that, for them, it is more of an organic condition. The growing reference to lifestyle with regard to health among the older children would indicate that they begin to become more aware of societal factors.

These studies illustrated the value of using drawings as a means of exploring children's understandings of health and illness and demonstrated how these were linked with their socio-cultural context. However, the studies were largely descriptive and primarily concluded by describing two broad categories of children's understandings of health—biomedical and psychosocial. They did not explicitly consider the underlying dynamics of the children's understandings or the context within which they constructed their views on health and illness. Several of the studies referred to the importance of harmony as central to social representations of health. This was also identified in subsequent studies with adults (see Herzlich's work in Chap. 5).

4.3 Gen Xers in England, 1970–1985

Moving into adolescence and early adulthood, young people begin to gain greater independence. Several studies have explored how this is reflected in their health-related practices and their understandings of health and illness. In 1950, over 80% of adult men and 40% of adult women in the UK smoked cigarettes. Following the growing evidence of the link between smoking and lung cancer (Doll & Hill, 1952), there was a sustained campaign to reduce its prevalence. However, by 1970, the prevalence of smoking among men was still 70%, and among women, it had risen to 50% (Peto et al., 2000).

In 1971, following the growing public debate about smoking among children and adolescents, a study of smoking among primary school children in the English Midlands was initiated by a public health physician, Beulah Bewley (Bewley, 2016). The original study was a questionnaire survey of over 7000 10- to 11½-year-old children on their smoking habits and perceptions of smoking and smokers. It was found that while 6.9% of boys and 2.9% of girls reported regular smoking, a further 36% of boys and 20% of girls had experimented with smoking (Bewley et al., 1973).

Following these studies of children, Bewley initiated a large longitudinal survey of teenage smoking, which began in 1974 and continued until 1978. Each year, for five years, a large sample of teenagers answered a questionnaire about their smoking practices and attitudes (e.g., Banks et al., 1978; Johnson et al., 1981). This survey confirmed that adolescence was the period during which smoking habits became established and that, by the time they reached 16 years, the majority of teenagers had tried smoking, and about one quarter were smoking regularly.

This large longitudinal study described the various correlates of smoking during adolescence. Smoking was more common among boys from working-class homes whose parents smoked. When I became involved in the research, an analysis of the comments written by the teenagers on the questionnaires helped to expand our understanding of the adoption of smoking (Murray, 1983). It was closely tied to gender representations and the process of identity formation. The young teenage boys from working-class homes sought to stress their masculinity through their physical prowess and adoption of working-class habits such as smoking. One theme was that of independence. As one teenage boy said: 'If you want to smoke then you can if you like. What you do with your private life is your own concern, it should not be controlled by others but left to the individual [...] If you want to smoke then you should be allowed to. Life is what you make of it, not what is made for you'. A teenage girl had a similar view: 'So what if people do smoke? There's hardly anything you can do about it! I want to start smoking in the future and I wouldn't thank you for interfering or getting smoking banned'. Among these working-class adolescents, smoking was represented as a symbol of independence and adulthood, which they were attempting to integrate into their own identity.

In 1981, an extension of this study followed the original cohort of teenagers investigated into early adulthood. This time, the questionnaire survey was complemented by a detailed interview with a sample of the participants. This provided an opportunity to explore the everyday lives of the young people and their views on health, illness and smoking (Murray & Jarrett, 1985; Murray et al., 1988). Theoretically, the study was based upon Harré and Secord's (1972) ethogenic approach. This approach argued that people's social behaviour is governed by social rules and that people have the ability to give accounts of their actions. The challenge for the researcher is not only to obtain but also to critically interpret such accounts. Here, we will consider how they contribute to our understanding of social representations of health and illness.

The interview study took place in 1982 in a small industrial town in the English Midlands. This was a town with a long history of manufacturing and service industries, such that many of the young people expected to get a job in a local factory or office when they left school. However, this was the beginning of the de-industrialization of Britain, with many industries closing and unemployment rising. The 1980s was the period when Margaret Thatcher's Conservative government was in power, with its policies of privatization, deregulation, cuts in government funding and generalized attacks on organized labour. Unemployment in the UK peaked at 3.3 million (13%) in 1984, and among young people, there was anxiety about their future prospects. These young people have subsequently been termed members of Generation X, or Gen Xers. These are those who were born in the 15-year period (1965–1980) after the baby-boomers. They were particularly impacted by the economic and political turbulence facing British society in the 1980s. This was reflected in the popular music of the time. In 1981, the two-tone group *The Specials* topped the singles chart with *Ghost Town*, a rather morbid song about unemployment and deindustrialization. The following year, the song *Come on Eileen* by the group Dexy's Midnight Runners topped the popular music charts, followed in 1983 by *Relax* by Frankie Goes to Hollywood. Both of these high-energy songs exhorted young people to get out and enjoy life despite the economic uncertainty. It was during this period that the study was conducted.

A sample of young people who had participated in the original school survey was contacted by mail and invited to participate in a follow-up interview. These interviews took place in their homes, often in the evening when the young people had returned from work. The interviews were informal and sought a narrative account of their lives at home, work and leisure, as well as their use of cigarettes in these different settings.

A total of 49 young people were interviewed, of which 28 were male and 21 were female. Most of the interviews were with working-class youth, reflecting the composition of the town. Many of these young working-class men and women had left school at 16 years and had entered various manual and clerical occupations. The interviews were transcribed and reviewed to explore their representations of health, illness and smoking, as well as the different contexts within which smoking occurred. The analysis deliberately aimed to place their understandings of health and illness within their immediate social setting. This is illustrated with extracts from the interviews.

In 1984, a large-scale postal survey was conducted with the young people who had participated in the school-based survey six years earlier. These young people were originally residents of the administrative county where they had attended school. Various strategies were used to trace these young people, and 4778 (63.3% of the targeted sample) ultimately completed the survey. The questionnaire used was based on the information collected in the interview study. Of these young people, 51% were female, and the others were male. One-third of the women were married, as were 17% of the men. A total of 74% of the men were in full-time employment, as were 67% of the women. Of those who were still single, most still lived with their parents.

Here, we integrate these two sources of information about young people's views on health and illness. Their social representations of health were anchored within their everyday lives and related to issues of gender and social class.

Social life: On leaving school, most of the young adults gained employment in local industry. This was a challenging but exciting time for them. According to Levinson's (1978) theory of social development, this was the period of transition to early adulthood when they were entering the world of work with older adults, developing social and romantic relationships and separating from their parents. The young people talked about gaining independence from their parents, developing new relationships, and their plans for the future. Most led an active social life, which centred around the pub, but many were also engaged in sporting and other leisure activities. It is within this context that we can begin to understand their social representations of health and illness.

Health: The primary dimension in their social representations of health was *fitness* and the *ability to carry on with everyday activities.* In existentialist terms, this could be described as a 'doing' definition of health and would suggest that the young people *anchored* health in everyday activity. Almost every male referred to fitness when asked to define health. For example, one young man defined health as 'being basically sound, y'know, fit', while another defined it as 'a reasonable fitness both mentally and physically'. The young women used this term less frequently, although it was still the most popular definition of health for them. For example, one young woman defined health as 'being as fit as you possibly can be'.

Both the young men and women usually extended their definition of fitness to emphasize the active dimension. Fitness was perceived as the ability to perform tasks—it was not exceptional; rather, it was normal. As one young woman said: 'To be able to run up the stairs without having to pant at the top … to be able to go to places, do things you want to do, and not be able to tell when you've done it'.

Several of the young men, in their attempts to underline the normality of health, distinguished athleticism from fitness. Being athletic was not considered normal. One young man explained the difference:

> I'm super fit. I mean I'm pretty big here, but I can sort of look after myself. I can do a day's work without feeling too tired, y'know. I'd say I'm fit enough to do my job. I wouldn't say I'm a sportsman. I'm not athletic. I'm fairly healthy. I wouldn't say I'm, y'know, an athletic person but I'm sort of fit enough to cope with every day needs that I need to do like.

Another young man tried to differentiate between normal health and athleticism, although he termed the latter fitness. As he said: 'Healthy's easy really—just go through the routine of eating, going to sleep. But to keep fit, that's running, squash, sports in general'. There was this association between normality and fitness for both the young men and women, but you could do certain things to enhance your fitness and help improve your standing with your peers.

The other main dimension of health was the *state of a person's body* and *mind*. In existentialist terms, this was more a 'having' definition of health. In this way they *objectified* health as something that they had as part of their person. One young man defined health as 'a situation where there's nothing physically or mentally wrong with you'. Another was more expansive:

> I suppose it depends on, y'know, your body an' that. Err, I know some illnesses can be caused by the job you're doing and that but most of it depends on how your body's built and that, y'know, if you're immune to certain things.

Table 4.1 Personal definition of health

	(n)	*Carry on with usual activities (%)*	*Fitness (%)*	*State of body (%)*	*State of mind (%)*
Male	(2272)	37.9	29.2	23.8	9.2
Female	(1203)	37.4	23.9	24.7	14.0

Source Murray et al. (1988)

In the survey, the young people were asked to indicate which of four definitions 'best describes health'. Table 4.1 details the proportion preferring each definition of health, classified by their gender. The most popular definition was 'ability to carry on', followed by 'fitness', then 'state of body' and finally 'state of mind'. In general, more men than women preferred the 'fitness' definition, whereas more women than men preferred the 'state of mind' definition. The latter difference reached statistical significance. Furthermore, the non-manual workers were consistently more likely than the manual workers to define health as a 'state of body', although this difference did not reach significance.

The definition of health preferred was related to both the gender and social class of the young adults. The young men's greater preference for 'fitness' as a definition reflected their greater concern about physical effectiveness. Strength and fitness were represented as the male ideal to which they aspired.

A main concern among the young men was physical prowess and the ability to handle oneself. Health was defined by fitness and strength. These were features that were needed both in the workplace and in their everyday lives. The young women used this definition less frequently than the young men did. The young women were more concerned with how they looked, such that gender differences in social representations of health defined health in terms of strength and fitness for men, while for women it was more about beauty and sociability (Murray & Jarrett, 1985). Health was *anchored* in their ability to do things in work and social relationships while it was also *objectified* in their bodies. For the young men, it was the ability to handle often strenuous work, and for the young women, it was more about their image to others, which was important in developing romantic relationships.

It was not uncommon for the young men to be involved in various sporting and athletic activities, which contributed to fitness and strength as well as providing companionship. The young women entered various routine manual workplaces where physical strength was less important. For them, social relationships were of prime importance. An important concern among these young women was looking good, having friends, attracting a partner, marriage and motherhood. The survey conducted in the following year found that 32.9% of the young women were married compared to 16.6% of the young men.

Health practices: These gender differences in social representations of health were apparent in their replies to the survey about health practices. The young men's health practices were particularly concerned with activities such as body-building and weight-training, which would aid the development of the ideal muscular male form. On the other hand, the young women preferred keep-fit classes and dieting. This agrees with the research conducted around the same time, suggesting that the self-concept of late adolescent boys was related to their physical effectiveness, whereas the self-concept of late adolescent girls was based on the assessment of their own physical attractiveness. In their study, Lerner and Karabenick (1974) reported that during late adolescence, girls were more concerned about their bodies' physical attractiveness, whereas boys were more concerned about physical effectiveness.

The character of the young men's health practices was also related to the fitness definition of health. There were many examples of these male fitness activities. This was the case for both smokers and non-smokers. One young male smoker said: 'I march miles and miles. I cycle ... That's why I don't buy a car ... If you buy a car you get lazy'. Meanwhile, a young male non-smoker added: 'I do press-ups every night and every morning ... When I'm at university I go jogging every day'.

The young women also engaged in physical exercise activities, although to a lesser extent than they used diet or weight control. It was noticeable that their exercises were not strenuous but more of the keep-fit type, which are also related to weight control. One young woman's comments were typical: 'I exercise and that's about it. Just sort of keep-fit things, y'know, touching me toes ... I used to go jogging a lot. I've packed up a lot now though. I don't have time'. Their interest in keep-fit activities was part of their concern with body image.

For most of the young women, health maintenance meant diet and weight control—essential for maintaining the ideal female shape. One young woman said: 'I try to have a balanced diet which is also basically to do with watching your weight but it's still to do with your health as well'. Smoking was seen by some of these young women as an aid to weight control—an aid to being healthy. As a young female smoker said: '[Smoking] stopped me biting me nails and it made me lose a lot of weight as well'.

Related to the definition of health as a state of mind was the view that health maintenance was partly psychological. As one young woman said: 'Get out and enjoy themselves, don't let things get them down. Just take life as it comes, I'd say, but some people take it too seriously. They worry over things that aren't worth worrying about'. The young men had a similar view. As one young man said: 'It's a very mental matter. It's a lot to do with the mind. In some ways if you try and stay alert and keep happy you're probably a bit more resilient.'

Illness: Illness was defined in terms of limitations on physical and social activities. For young men, illness meant interference with the ability to perform physical activities. For these young men, the emphasis was on strength. Consider this comment by one of the young male smokers:

> I like smoking and I don't care if it is rotting me insides. I don't feel any worse. I mean perhaps I might get out of puff running up the street a bit more but then again I'm not an athletic person. I'm more muscley for me job rather than run up and down the street every two minutes ... In the job I do I don't get out of puff but probably running up the road all day I'd get out of puff dead fast which someone else who doesn't smoke probably won't.

Similarly, for the young female smokers, the benefits of smoking in social settings outweighed concerns about its negative effects on their lives. For example, one young woman who had recently adopted smoking was aware of the ill-effects it had on her life: '... before I could run ... before, when I was in the band I never smoked and then when I went back and started playing again, I get out of breath so easily'. However, smoking was important in her social life. The recreational life of these young people centred on the pub, where smoking was an important aid to social interaction. Smoking was not banned in British bars until 2007. Illness was defined in terms of destruction of ability to perform everyday activities.

The primary cause of illness was *way-of-life*. Since activity was central to health, those factors which restricted activity were the primary cause of ill-health. Consider the case of the young man who was a seasonal fairground worker. During the summer, he worked in a coastal resort and felt very healthy. But during the winter months, when he was unemployed in Peakside, he felt some inertia setting in:

> I was fit as hell when I was at Bellstown, y'know. I lost a lot of weight and what not and built me muscles up – it's all cutting and scraping, woodwork, concrete. Down there I don't mind [running] along the sea and back. I don't mind that a bit ... but now I've come back here and I haven't got no job or doing anything. I've put on a pound and that, but that's what happens – you get it in the winter, you lose it in the summer.

Besides the way-of-life, there was also the issue of *inheritance*. This was the individual reserve of health that the young adult had inherited. As one young man said:

> I suppose it depends on y'know, your body and that. I know some illnesses can be caused by the job you're doing and that, but most of it depends on how your body's built and that, if you're immune to certain things.

In addition, they noted that the body generally deteriorates with age, but also that consequent reduced activity could lead to ill-health:

> Well eventually you get ... I mean ... I don't see it matters when you're young but when you start getting older you just stay about in the house all day eating and smoking and it can cause damage to your heart.

There was also a reference to *psychological factors* as a cause. This view was more common among the young women:

> ...it can sometimes be your state of mind, apart from the obvious diseases that make you sick. How you feel. If you feel low and depressed it can make you feel ill in different ways or if you feel happy and confident then you feel better.

Social class, gender and health: The young people anchored their representations of health and illness in social and physical activity. The young men, in particular, referred to physical activity as the prime definition of health. It was also a necessity for health. Many of the young people participated in active physical pursuits to maintain their level of health and fitness. For the young women, health activity was mainly in terms of keep-fit activities and diet. Besides being part of health maintenance, these activities were also aimed at maintaining physical attractiveness.

Social representations of health were linked with representations of social class and gender. The dominant representation of masculinity among the young people in this largely working-class community was in terms of strength/fitness, whereas for femininity, it was more in terms of elegance/beauty. Health for these young men was represented in terms of muscular strength and physical fitness, and activities that could increase these capacities, such as strength training and sporting activities, were preferred. Smoking was accepted as long as it did not interfere with these capacities. Indeed, smoking could even be seen as an indication of strength if it did not immediately impair everyday health. Health for the young women was more in terms of an elegance/attractiveness version of bodily potency, and activities such as keep-fit and dieting that could enhance it were favoured.

Illness was the loss of activity. This could be brought about by changes in social circumstances, but the young people strove to overcome these restrictions despite the larger social challenges. Herzlich (1973) found a similar representation in her study of adults. She noted that the link between inactivity and illness led to the representation acquiring a particular function: 'Through it, by refusal or justification of the inactivity of the invalid, the subject's attempt to relate himself to society as a whole finds expression' (p. 137). In our case, the young people maintained health and avoided illness through physical activity and thus maintained their role in society.

A theme that ran through these accounts was identity and the struggle for independence. Pitti (2017) found that representations of attaining adulthood in Western society are largely framed in terms of achieving independence from parents, while continued dependence on parents reflects a delay in the transition to adulthood. There were two main dimensions in the GenXers' social representations of adulthood. One was *independence-dependence,* and the other was *solitary-community*. Taking these two dimensions as orthogonal, the favoured quadrant was independence/community, where young people could display their adulthood in the company of friends. In working-class neighbourhoods smoking was an intrinsic part of membership in this quadrant. The extent to which a person could achieve independence was associated with health, whereas dependency was seen as a form of illness. In the 1980s, many young people managed to leave the family home, but this was not so easy for the next generation.

4.4 Millennials in England 2010–2020

Twenty-five years later, things had changed dramatically for young people in Britain. In the 1970s and 1980s, most young people left school, sought employment and moved out of the family home in their late teens or early twenties, whereas by the 2000s, more young people were in education or training, and movement out of the home and the gaining of independence was delayed (Coleman, 2000). The decline of the manufacturing industry in Britain had a particularly negative impact on young men, who found it more difficult to gain employment. Young women's educational performance began to exceed that of young men, and they were more likely to go on to higher education. The early 2000s witnessed the global financial crisis of 2007–2008, which impacted the already limited job opportunities for young people. There were riots involving young people in many urban settings across Britain. A particular feature of the music scene among young people was the rise of Grime and Drill music, with jagged sounds and lyrics about the precariousness of young people's lives, with songs like *Fix Up, Look Sharp* by Dizzee Rascal.

In this difficult climate, the so-called Millennials (born between 1981 and 2000) began to smoke and drink less. The prevalence of smoking declined substantially among young people, but this was followed by a sustained increase in the use of electronic cigarettes (Public Health England, 2020). Smoking became more common among young middle-class women (Buss et al., 2024). New health issues began to develop. According to surveys, there was an overall decline in satisfaction with health and evidence of increasing anxiety and depression among young women, while suicide rates increased among young men (Department of Education, 2022).

A series of studies explored how these young people talked about smoking in their lives. Although the young people in these studies did not talk explicitly about health, they provided some indication of their social representations of health. In one study by Grogan et al. (2009), focus groups were held with a sample of young male and female smokers and non-smokers aged 16–24 years in a northern English city. The focus groups considered motivations for smoking but also physical appearance issues. Previous research had indicated that young women associated youth with beauty (Grogan, 2008). While young men were becoming more concerned with physical appearance, they still appeared reluctant to admit appearance concerns (Grogan & Richards, 2002; Hargreaves & Tiggermann, 2006).

Talking about sport and physical activities was a socially acceptable way for young men to talk about their bodies (Grogan, 2008).

Thematic analysis of the interview transcripts about smoking identified a core category of 'Youth and Beauty'. *Looking young* (wrinkle-free and attractive) was the ideal image for these young people, although *being young* (inexperienced and immature) was not perceived positively. More detailed analysis of this core category revealed that, for the young people, smoking was an indicator of maturity but also a means for women to keep thin. Being thin was linked to both youth and attractiveness. However, non-smokers were concerned about the negative effects of smoking on skin and teeth, making them sexually unattractive. The male non-smokers were particularly concerned that smoking would yellow their skin and teeth, which was linked to looking unclean and being sexually unattractive. This reference to cleanliness, rather than beauty, was a means for men to avoid seeming overly concerned about physical attractiveness.

Research into young adults' perceptions of e-cigarettes found that young people considered them less harmful than cigarettes and, indeed, an aid to smoking cessation. They were also viewed as an important tool for identification with a valued social group. In a study conducted in the north of England, an open-ended questionnaire was administered to a sample of adults ranging in age from 18 to 65 years (Ranjit et al., 2021). A grounded theory analysis of the responses identified four main categories to summarize their responses. The most important of these was social context, which emphasized that the use of e-cigarettes or vaping occurred in social situations and was a fun activity. Another theme specifically addressed the health aspects of vaping, which was seen as a healthy alternative to smoking. Health was described as enjoying social life while not endangering one's health through smoking.

The third study involved individual interviews about vaping with five men and seven women aged 23–55 years in a northern English city (Wilson et al., 2022). Thematic analysis of the interview transcripts identified three themes. The first theme was concerned with social influence and the role that others played in the adoption of vaping. This is similar to previous findings that vaping was considered a fun activity. The second theme concerned the public representation of vaping as a safe alternative to cigarette smoking. The third theme concerned addiction, particularly vaping as a safe alternative to smoking.

Together, this research on smoking and vaping extended the earlier research on smoking among young people and their social representations of health. The core social representation of health among the young people was concerned with physical appearance rather than fitness—more ***having*** than ***doing***. There were clear gender differences, with the young women emphasizing the value of smoking as an aid to weight control, but among young men, there remained an apprehension about excessive concern with beauty.

In addition, as they moved into the twenty-first century, the Millennials faced a range of new social challenges. For example, more young people were continuing in education or training, and with the increasing cost of housing, they were finding it more difficult to leave the family home. This, in some ways, extended youth culture as the pathway into the more independent lifestyle of adulthood was delayed. A major challenge faced by young people was related to changes in gender roles and expectations. There is also the problem of gaining independence from the family. Several studies have considered the impact of these challenges on social representations of health among young adults.

An additional issue is the retrospective anchoring of smoking in earlier times, which reflects the trans-generational impact on contemporary youth culture of previous generations. The French novelist Michel Houellebecq, in *Les Particules élémentaires* (1998), has argued that the individualistic and self-seeking culture of the sixties has contributed to modern sexual and social alienation among young people (Michallat, 2007; Michallat & Tinker, 2007). A reflection of this is the apparent contemporary nostalgia among young people for the carefree attitude of their parents and grandparents. Nostalgia was originally a reaction to difficult times and was considered an illness. Now, it is considered an emotion that conveys dissatisfaction with the modern world and a yearning for times past (Arnold-Forster, 2024; Sedikides & Wildschut, 2023). Young people look back to a time when you could enjoy guilt-free smoking and live in an era without indoor smoking restrictions. Modern films often portray people smoking as a symbolic nod to these halcyon days (Rufo, 2024). Smoking has become anchored in those supposedly good times.

4.5 Millennials in France 2010–2020

Since the end of the Second World War, the role of women in French and other Western societies has changed dramatically. Traditionally, France was very much a patriarchal society. It was not until 1944 that women won the right to vote. In 1949, Simone de Beauvoir published her famous book entitled *Le Deuxième Sexe* (*The Second Sex,* de Beauvoir, 1954), which clearly articulated the sex-gender distinction with its famous phrase, '*On ne naît pas femme, on le deviant*', which has been translated as 'One is not born a woman but becomes a woman'. Woman is socially and historically constructed and constructs herself as a woman. Since then, women in France have steadily combatted social oppression and asserted their rights. During the 1960s and 1970s, the pace of change increased. In 1965, women gained the right to work without their husband's consent. In 1967, contraception was legalized and in 1975, abortion in certain circumstances was approved.

However, the growth of neoliberalism in the 1980s in many Western countries threatened this movement towards greater equality. Women continued to mobilize for greater rights, and towards the end of the twentieth century, there was a rise in militancy about violence against women as well as sustained debate about changing gender roles (Allwood & Wadia, 2002).

The early 2000s was a period of sustained discussion in French society about sex and gender, about equality at work and at home and about the composition of the family (Perreau & Scott, 2017). Popular youth songs at that time included *Toutes les Femmes de ta Vie* [All the Women in Your Life] by the all-woman group L5, which celebrated the diversity and strength of women, and *Garçon* [Boy] by Koxie, which tackled the issue of street harassment and promoted gender equality.

In this period, Marie-Anastasie Aim and her colleagues in Aix-en-Provence conducted a series of studies exploring young people's social representations of health and gender in France. They noted that, in discussing health issues, the young people also talked about their social relationships, expectations, and social identities.

In one of these studies (Aim et al., 2020) focus groups were conducted with young men and women (both single and mixed-gender) to discuss their views on health and health practices. The aim was to explore how these young people intertwined their discussions of health and gender. The focus group transcripts were subjected to thematic content analysis and group dynamic analysis, and in their analyses, they adopted a discursive and socio-cultural approach.

The majority of the young men and women emphasized the similarity in their representations of health and in their health practices. They also referred to the changes in gender identity. For example, one young man said, 'It's more to do with trends. Out of a concern to belong to certain social groups'. However, he also added, 'Men and women's brains don't work in the same way' (p. 1908). This perceived gender difference was related to the gender composition of the focus groups. While the unisex groups tempered differences, the mixed groups referred to differences, e.g., 'Being women we're going to think about certain things; they, as men, will think about other things'. These differences were related to historical factors. For example, one woman said, 'In previous generations men and women had completely different ideas about good health'. Previously they were concerned about health at home and their children, whereas 'today, women have to, they have to do sport like men'. The perceived reduction of gender differences encouraged the women to behave more like men.

Both men and women agreed that women would be more accepting of mental healthcare, while men would rely on physicality. Men would be more risk-taking, whereas women would adopt a more cautious, preventive stance regarding their health. As one man said about women: 'A little more sensible, yeah. They have to protect themselves' (p. 1909).

An important distinction was made regarding perceptions of differences in men's and women's bodies. For women, it was felt there was a societal requirement to have both a healthy and beautiful body. As one woman said: 'There's an image of women that they have to be slim, have a beautiful body, all that' (p. 1910). Women were also expected to consider their potential maternal role. As one man said: 'In any case she carries the child for nine months, so it's generally women who are most concerned because it's about the child's health' (p. 1910).

It was agreed that there was what was described as an 'imperative of health'. This required both self-monitoring and work. The perceived different health demands were justified by the sex differences in physiology. Thus, the reason why women were expected to be more concerned about taking care of their bodies was that they were potential mothers. Aim et al. 2020 summarized this process: 'By invoking "biological health", biopolitics (Foucault, 1979) can thus function in a framework that naturalizes the social' (p. 1913). However, the young people were aware of these justificatory processes and engaged in debate to challenge the social expectations. Thus, the social representations of health engaged with the broader sociocultural differences in gender role expectations.

By referring to biology, participants 'naturalized' gender differences regarding health. It was felt that women would be more inclined to accept mental healthcare, whereas men would be more physically resistant and prone to taking risks. Women were perceived to have a 'natural' preventive stance because they could be potential victims of aggression.

An important distinction was made regarding what was described as aesthetics and the reproductive female body. The societal requirement to maintain a healthy body was a more significant issue for women. The size of the investment in the feminine aesthetic was described as being more important. Female biological characteristics (e.g., periods, pregnancy) anchored feminine health within the mother's health category. As one young woman said: 'Women take care of their children ... the mother has more need to know about illness'.

Women's health is connected to family life, both now and in the future, whereas men's health is thought to be more 'personal'. The young people described men as autonomous, strong and tough. Women were more often described as fragile, having a certain ease in expressing their feelings, and seeking help. It was felt that feminine health identity was characterized by a self-monitoring requirement: 'We're told "be careful", we're told all through middle school "use protection"'.

This study focused on how social representations are discussed and maintained in everyday social interaction. These young people were actively engaged in a process of enacting social expectations. The social representations contained mixed views on health and gender, which they negotiated in their everyday lives. The original view of social representations was that, although it may contain contradictions, it is still relatively cohesive and stable. In this study, there was a certain tension with the changing views on gender, but these were accommodated in the young people's social interaction.

Young people are surrounded by popular images of gender in newspapers, magazines, social media and various art forms. A popular genre of literature for young people is graphic novels and comics. In France, the *bande dessinée* (BD) is an extremely popular genre. The images presented in such literature are particularly important for understanding social representations of gender and health. A study of gender representations in BDs found that historically, women have always been represented in a subservient position in these publications (MacLeod, 2021). In a study of representations of *Wonder Woman* in superhero comics conducted by a Brazilian team, it was found that although *Wonder Woman* was an active hero, in order to maintain her femininity, her feminine aspects, such as her hair and body shape, were accentuated, while more masculine aspects, such as physical strength, were portrayed mildly (Guimaraes et al., 2024). In another study of superhero comics in the United States, Carolyn Cocca (Cocca, 2014) noted that 'feminine signifiers are emphasized to the point of parody, with exaggerated features such as sexy hair even underwater and an exaggerated curvature of the upper body that accentuates the breasts and creates an hourglass effect on the hips'. Such images contribute to the focus on glamourous physical appearance in women's social representations of health.

4.6 Young Homeless People in Germany 2000s

As the world entered the twenty-first century, more challenges faced the Western world. One of the challenges facing youth in gaining independence has been finding suitable living accommodation. An associated problem is that of homelessness. It has been estimated that in England alone, 282,000 single people, couples and families were homeless or threatened with homelessness in 2020/21 (Watts et al., 2022). This includes people who engage in 'rough sleeping' (on the street, in doorways, in parks, etc.), people temporarily living in shelters or people living in the homes of friends. The most important cause of this is the lack of affordable housing, but certain factors may exacerbate the likelihood of homelessness. These include relationship breakdowns, violent or abusive relationships, mental and physical health problems, along with a lack of income. The experience of homelessness can increase the extent of threat to the homeless person, with many reporting being victims of violence.

A study in Germany explored the social representations of health among homeless adolescents (Flick & Rohnsch, 2007). In this study, a sample of 24 homeless adolescents participated in an episodic interview about what health meant to them and what their experiences of health and health problems were. The adolescents mainly referred to family conflicts as the primary reason why they ended up homeless. Their representations of health were categorized into four categories: Health as physical and mental well-being, health as a result of specific practices, health as the absence of illness and health as functionality. Few of the adolescents defined health solely in terms of the absence of illness but rather described it in more social terms: 'when they say that health also means to remain capable of acting and to be integrated in a satisfying environment' (p. 742). Since this definition was not that different from other adolescents, it was suggested that these homeless adolescents did not consider their living conditions important.

However, when asked about their own experiences of health, the majority of these young adolescents were not optimistic. Their replies were organized into four categories: Health as a distant ideal, denial of health problems, health as relative and health as reality. The most common experience was that of health being an ideal that was out of reach. Their homelessness meant that while they stressed the importance of social integration in their definition of health, this was not something that they felt they could achieve.

This study further illustrates how the social representations of health are intertwined with everyday experiences and the opportunity to exercise agency, rather than an acceptance of their situation. The struggle for independence was confused because, for some, leaving a violent or abusive home was an attempt to gain independence rather than remaining constrained by a threatening home-life.

4.7 Embodied Social Representations

Social representations of health and illness are not fixed but evolve as we develop and encounter new challenges in our everyday lives. Physical activity and the body are central to the lives of young people. This is reflected in the primacy given to these factors in social representations of health. The social representation of health is shaped not just by social engagement but also by the physical engagement of the body. This idea draws upon the concept of embodied cognition and Merleau-Ponty's phenomenology. According to embodied cognition, the body is actively involved in shaping our understanding of the world (Varela et al., 2017). Similarly, Merleau-Ponty emphasized that we are inseparable from our bodies, which are enmeshed in our social world. We are physical beings, and the ability of our bodies to function effectively is reflected in our social representation, which is tested in our social and physical interaction with the environment. It is a circular or dynamic relationship between the inner and outer. As Merleau-Ponty (1942) said, 'The relations between the organism and its environment are not relations of linear causality, but of circular causality' (Merleau-Ponty, [1942] 1965).

Although Merleau-Ponty emphasized the centrality of the physical body in human perception, it is still possible to accentuate the social standing of our bodily form through such means as exercise, clothing and cosmetics, but also through drugs and surgery. The body is not just a means of physical activity but also of strength and beauty. These issues become increasingly important as young people develop an understanding of their place in the world and of health and illness. Their understandings are located in both their everyday relationships and the broader socio-cultural expectations. Their social representations are also embedded in their everyday activities. As Herzlich (1973) said: 'A child seems not to grasp what illness [and health] is nor to understand its future significance in his life: he has to learn to locate his experience in a framework of social explanations and rules' (p. 1).

Young people are generally healthy, and it is not surprising that they consider health as the norm. It is normal to be healthy and to get on with your life. As they grow into early adulthood, the quest is to break away from family ties and to establish new relationships. However, as we enter the twenty-first century, for many young people, this has become more difficult. There are gender differences in their life expectations and in their social representations of health. These gender differences are enmeshed in the sustained cultural changes in Britain and elsewhere.

The social representations of gender are involved in young people's identity. Boys and young men emphasize the importance of strength in their understanding of health, while for girls and young women, it is more concerned with sociability and beauty. However, this gender difference is not fixed but is negotiated in everyday social interaction. It is a social representation that is related to the identity of these young people, who are gaining independence from their families and developing relationships with others. However, limitations on their ability to gain independence, due to political and economic challenges as well as the impact of cultural changes in gender definitions, are reflected in their social representations of health.

Another way of understanding these changes is to consider female-male as a key thematic concept. Marková (2023) suggested, 'female-male as a thematic concept [which] focuses on transformations of interdependent dialogical oppositions, for example, motherhood/fatherhood, rights/duties, biological equalities/inequalities' (p. 168). In the case of health/illness, female health was described in terms of attractiveness and elegance, which could be promoted by diet and keep-fit exercises. Male health was characterized by strength and vigour which could be promoted by exercise and sporting activities. While mental health was consistently considered an aspect of representations of health and illness, managing mental health issues was regarded as more problematic among men. Several studies have reported the higher rate of mental health problems and suicide among young men (Coleman, 2000).

At the socio-historical level, there was evidence of a shift in social representations of health from one that placed emphasis on doing to one that was more about having. The doing was concerned with the ability to perform certain activities, while the having was the possession of certain qualities. This reflected the broader consumerist ethos of contemporary Western culture (Portin, 2020). In this stage of neoliberalism, not only goods and services but our very identity has become marketable. In this climate, health becomes something that can be purchased through the wearing of sports clothing and membership in gyms (Gould & Gould, 2001). For many young people, access to these health markers is often outside their reach, leading to frustration and anxiety and the increasing reference to mental health issues in social representations of health and illness. The doing orientation seemed to be less important in representations of health among millennials.

Another important factor is the decline in public venues where young people can easily socialize and where social representations of health are debated and challenged. Oldenburg (1989) and others (e.g., Oldenburg & Brissett, 1982) have commented on the deleterious impact of the decline of the so-called 'third place', such as bars and clubs, in Western society, where informal socializing can take place outside the home and work settings. In Britain, this is reflected in the decline in the number of pubs, which are the traditional venues for socializing, especially among young men (Roberts & Townshend, 2013). Instead, millennials have turned to the internet. In this location, understandings of health and illness are defined less by physical performance and more by mental agility.

Changes in gender roles and expectations were reflected in the changes in representations of health. Among young women, there was tension between beauty and the ability to perform like a man in sporting and other activities. Among men, there was tension between physicality and awareness of emotional health. These tensions were negotiated in everyday social interaction. An important absence in the content of these young people's social representations of health was the discussion of sexuality. This was surprising in view of the importance of relationships among this age group. It may be that young people consider sexual relationships as something separate from health or that it is a private matter they prefer not to discuss. This was the muting of discussion of this more private domain of health.

References

Aim, M.-A., Lelaurain, S., Khatmi, N., Fonte, D., Bovina, I., & Dany, L. (2020). 'Similar but different': Social representations of health according to gender for French youth. *Journal of Health Psychology*, 25(12), 1905–1916.

Allwood, G., & Wadia, K. (2002). French feminisms: National and international perspectives. *Modern & Contemporary France*, 10(2), 211–223.

Arnold-Forster, A. (2024). *Nostalgia: A history of a dangerous emotion*. Picador.

Banks, M. H., Bewley, B. R., Bland, J. M., Dean, J. R., & Pollard, V. M. (1978). A long-term study of smoking by secondary schoolchildren. *Archives of Disease in Childhood*, 53, 12–19.

Bewley, B. (2016). *Beulah Bewley. My life as a woman and doctor*. Silverwood.

Bewley, B. R., Halil, T., & Snaith, A. H. (1973). Smoking by primary schoolchildren: Prevalence and associated respiratory symptoms. *British Journal of Preventive and Social Medicine*, 27, 150–153.

Bibace, R., & Walsh, M. E. (1980). Development of children's concepts of illness. *Pediatrics*, 66(6), 912–917.

Birns, B. (1972). Piaget and Wallon: Two giants of unequal visibility. *International Journal of Mental Health*, 1(4), 24–28.

Buss, V., West, R., Kock, L., & Brown, J. (2024). Annual trends on smoking in England from the smoking toolkit study. *Annual findings—Graphs—smoking in England*. https://smokinginengland.info/graphs/annual-findings.

Carey, S. (1985). *Conceptual change in childhood*. MIT Press.

Cocca, C. (2014). The 'Broke Back Test': A quantitative and qualitative analysis of portrayals of women in mainstream superhero comics, 1993–2013. *Journal of Graphic Novels and Comics*, 5(4), 411–428.

Coleman, J. (2000). Young people in Britain at the beginning of a new century. *Children & Society*, 14, 230–242.

Department of Education (2022). *State of the nation 2021: children and young people's wellbeing. Research report*. UK Government Social Research.

Doll, R., & Hill, A. B. (1952). A study of the aetiology of carcinoma of the lung. *BMJ*, 2, 1271–1286.

Duveen, G. (2001a). Representations, identities and resistance. In K. Deaux & G. Philogène (Eds.), *Representations of the social*. Blackwell.

Eiser, C. (1989). Children's concepts of illness: Towards an alternative to the "Stage" approach. *Psychology and Health*, 3(2), 93–101.

Eiser, C., Eiser, J. R., & Lang, J. (1989). Scripts in children's reports of medical events. *European Journal of Psychology of Education*, 4, 377–384.

Flick, U., & Rohnsch, G. (2007). Idealization and neglect: Health concepts of homeless adolescents. *Journal of Health Psychology*, 12(5), 737–749.

Foucault, M. (1979). *Naissance de la Biopolitique: Cours Au Collège de France*. Seuil.

Gould, N., & Gould, E. (2001). Health as a consumption object: Research notes and preliminary investigation. *International Journal of Consumer Studies*, 25, 90–101.

Grogan, S. (2008). *Body image: Understanding body dissatisfaction among men, women and children* (2nd Ed.). Taylor and Francis.

Grogan, S., Fry, G., Gough, B., & Conner, M. (2009). Smoking to stay thin or giving up to save face? Young men and women talk about appearance concerns and smoking. *British Journal of Health Psychology*, 14, 175–186.

Grogan, S., & Richards, H. (2002). Body image: Focus groups with boys and men. *Men and Masculinities*, 4, 219–233.

Guimaraes, L. E., Do Nascimento, A. R. A., Da Silva Costa, L. C., & De Oliveira, S. M. F. (2024). Femininity in superhero comics: A study of social representations. *Papers on Social Representations*, 33(1), 5.1–5.23.

Hargreaves, D., & Tiggermann, M. (2006). 'Body image is for girls': A qualitative study of boys' body image. *Journal of Health Psychology*, 11, 567–577.

Harré, R., & Secord, P. F. (1972). *The explanation of social behaviour*. Blackwell.

Herzlich, C. (1973). *Health and illness: A social psychological analysis*. Academic Press (Original work published 1969 as *Santé et Maladie: Analyse d'une Réprésentation Sociale*, Paris: Mouton).

Houellebecq. M. (1998). *Les particules élémentaires*. Flammarion.

Johnson, M. R. D., Murray, M., Bewley, B. R., & Clyde, D. C. (1981). Social class, parents, children and smoking. *Bulletin of the International Union Against Tuberculosis*, 57, 258–262.

Jovchelovitch, S., Priego-Hernández, J., & Glăveanu, V.-P. (2013). Constructing social worlds: Culture and socio-economic context in the development of children's representations of the public sphere. *Culture & Psychology*, 19(3), 323–347.

Jutras, S., & Bisson, J. (1994). La conception de la santé chez des enfants de 5 à 12 ans. Quelques clés pour la promotion de la santé. *Sciences sociales et santé*, 12 (2), 5–37.

Jutras, S., Morin, P., Proulx, R., Vinay, M. C., Roy, E., & Routhier, L. (2003). Conception of wellness in families with a diabetic child. *Journal of Health Psychology*, 8(5), 573–586.

Jutras, S., Normandeau, S., Kalnins, I., & Morin, P. (1998). Mental health referents within children's health cognitions. *Canadian Journal of Community Mental Health*, 17(1), 21–35.

Lerner, R. M., & Karabenick, S. A. (1974). Physical attractiveness, body attitudes and self-concept in late adolescence. *Journal of Youth and Adolescence*, 3, 307–310.

Levinson, D. (1978). *The seasons of a man's life*. A.A. Knopf.

Lloyd, B., & Duveen, G. (1992). *Gender identities and education: The impact of starting school*. Harvester-Wheatsheaf.

MacLeod, C. (2021). *Invisible presence: The representation of women in French-language comics.* Intellect Books.
Marková, I. (2023). *The making of a dialogical theory: Social representations and communication.* Cambridge University Press.
Merleau-Ponty, M. (1965). *The structure of behaviour.* Methuen.
Michallet, W. (2007). Modern life is still rubbish. Houellebecq and the refiguring of 'reactionary' retro. *Journal of European Studies*, 37(3), 313–331.
Michallet, W., & Tinkler, C. (2007). Introduction. *Modern & Contemporary France*, 15(3), 255–259.
Mouratidi, P.-S., Bonoti, F., & Leondari, A. (2016). Children's perceptions of illness and health: An analysis of drawings. *Health Education Journal*, 75(4), 434–447.
Murray, M. (1983). The social context of smoking during adolescence. In W. F. Forbes, R. C. Frecker, & D. Nosbakken (Eds.), *Proceedings of the fifth world conference on smoking and health.* Ottawa: Canadian Council on Smoking and Health.
Murray, M., & Jarrett, L. (1985). Young people's perceptions of health, illness and smoking. *Health Education Journal*, 44, 18–22.
Murray, M., Jarrett, L., Swan, A. V., & Rumun, R. (1988). *Smoking among young adults.* Gower.
Nelson, K. (1986). *Event knowledge: Structure and function in development.* Erlbaum.
Normandeau, S., Kalnins, I., Jutras, S., & Hanigan, D. (1998). A description of 5- to 12-year old children's conception of health within the context of their daily life. *Psychology and Health*, 13, 883–896.
Oldenburg, R. (1989). *The great good place: cafs, coffee shops, bookstores, bars, hair salons and other hangouts at the heart of the community.* Paragon House.
Oldenburg, R., & Brissett, D. (1982). The third place. *Qualitative Sociology*, 5, 265–284.
Perreau, B., & Scott, J.W. (2017). *Les défis de la République: Genre, territoires, citoyenneté.* Presses de Sciences Po.
Peto, R., Darby, S., Deo, H., Whitley, E., & Doll, R. (2000). Smoking, smoking cessation, and lung cancer in the UK since 1950: Combination of national statistics with two case-control studies. *BMJ*, 321, 323.
Piaget, J. (1932). *The moral judgment of the child.* Harcourt, Brace.
Piko, B. F., & Bak, J. (2006). Children's perceptions of health and illness: Images and lay concepts in preadolescence. *Education Research*, 21(5), 643–653.
Pitti, I. (2017). What does being an adult mean? Comparing young people's and adults' representations of adulthood. *Journal of Youth Studies*, 20(9), 1225–1241.

Portin, F. (2020). Consumerism as a moral attitude: Defining consumerism through the works of Pope Francis, Cornel West, and William T. Cavanaugh. *Nordic Journal of Theology*, 74(1), 4–24.

Pridmore, P., & Bendelow, G. (1995). Images of health: Exploring beliefs of children using the 'draw-and-write' technique. *Health Education Journal*, 54, 473–488.

Public Health England (2020). *Smoking prevalence in young adults aged 18 to 34 years*. Smoking prevalence in young adults aged 18 to 34 years—GOV.UK. https://www.gov.uk/government/publications/smoking-prevalence-in-young-adults-aged-18-to-34-years

Ranjit, A., McCutchan, G., Brain, K., & Poole, R. (2021). "That's the whole thing about vaping, it's custom tasty goodness": A metaethnography of young adults' perceptions and experiences of e-cigarette use. *Substance Abuse Treatment, Prevention and Policy*, 16(1), 85.

Roberts, M., & Townshend, T. (2013). Young adults and the decline of the urban English pub: Issues for planning. *Planning Theory & Practice*, 14(4), 455–469.

Rufo, Y. (2024). 'Pack of cigs and a Bic lighter': Why are celebs glamorizing smoking again? *BBC News Online*, 3 November. Are celebs such as Charli XCX and Addison Rae making smoking 'cool' again? https://www.bbc.co.uk/news/articles/ce8dy5v1kpno

Sedikides, C., & Wildschut, T. (2023). The psychological, social and societal relevance of nostalgia. *Current Opinion in Psychology*, 52, 101609.

van der Veer, R. (1996). Henri Wallon's theory of early childhood development: The role of emotions. *Developmental Review*, 16(4), 364–390.

Varela, F. J., Thompson, E., & Rosch, E. (2017). *The embodied mind: Cognitive science and human experience*. MIT Press.

Watts, B., Bramley, G., Fitzpatrick, S., McMordie, L., Pawson, H., & Young, G. (2022). *The homeless monitor: Great Britain 2022*. Crisis.

Wilson, G. L., Keenan, J., Grogan, S., Porcellato, L., Powell, S., & Gee, I. (2022). An investigation of factors encouraging and deterring EC use: A thematic analysis of accounts from UK adults. *Psychology and Health*, 37(11), 1379–1395.

CHAPTER 5

Health and Illness Among Adults

Moving into adulthood presents a new series of opportunities and challenges, including different experiences of health and illness. The character of these experiences is dependent upon the socio-cultural and historical setting. Over the past 60 years, there have been a series of studies on social representations of health and illness in different contexts. This chapter considers studies conducted in several countries in Western Europe. Each of these studies was conducted in a different socio-cultural location and also incorporated certain theoretical and methodological innovations. The chapter examines the role of the different settings and research approaches.

5.1 Adulthood

Having survived the travails of adolescence and early adulthood, adulthood is often characterized as a period of consolidation. The characterization of the transition from youth into adulthood as smooth was shaped during the post-war period, which was a time of growing prosperity in Western society. Young people were expected to leave the parental home, gain employment, marry and have children (Blatterer, 2007). However, times have changed, and this transition is no longer so smooth.

M. Murray, *Social Representations, Health and Illness*,
https://doi.org/10.1007/978-3-031-98494-5_5

A study conducted in Italy in the 2010s found that there was substantial tension between the ideal adult role and the opportunities and expectations. In this study, interviews were conducted with both young adults and 'significant' adults about their life prospects (Pitti, 2017). It was found that the two main characteristics frequently associated with adulthood were responsibility and independence. Responsibility was concerned with the expectation that an adult could take responsibility not only for their children but also for their parents and even for others in society. Independence was concerned with increasing autonomy, especially from parents, and freedom in choosing roles and activities. However, while these may have been the expectations, changing demands in society meant that many young adults found it difficult to fulfil them. Additionally, changing identity and role demands meant that many of the younger adults resisted certain expectations about responsibilities and asserted greater independence. As one young woman said:

> An adult has to be independent, autonomous, not dependent on anyone. In my family, a classic Southern family, my mother doesn't work and asks for money from my father even to buy a t-shirt. This is inconceivable to me, really. Today adult women should be autonomous as men are: we are no more in the nineteenth century! (p. 1231).

Although both younger people and adults agreed that responsibility and independence were central characteristics of the ideal adulthood, many of the young people were frustrated by the seeming reluctance of many adults to fulfil these characteristics. The youth often accused the typical adult of lacking maturity and adopting a youthful lifestyle. Some pointed to the precarious nature of modern existence, with regard to work and marriage, which meant that adults found it difficult to be responsible and independent.

While there has been a general improvement in health in Western society since the Second World War, there remain substantial social class differences. For example, a report by the British Department of Health found that, despite 30 years of a National Health Service, people from more working-class backgrounds were more likely to develop various health problems and to die earlier than people from more middle-class backgrounds (Townsend & Davidson, 1982). Subsequent reports have confirmed the continuing and extensive nature of this social class differential in health (e.g., Finch et al., 2023). Further, although the difference in the life expectancy of men and women has increased, men are still more likely to die earlier. These differences in health experiences are reflected in the different understandings of health and illness in different societies.

5.2 Adults in 1960s and 1970s France

Up until the Second World War, France had been primarily a rural society, but this changed in the years afterwards that was a period of rapid urbanization. The population of the country increased dramatically from 40 million in 1946 to 52 million in 1975. This population increase was due partly to the decline in infant mortality and the increase in life expectancy, but also to the rise in immigration from the former colonies. The influence of rural France declined as the country became more of an urban society. This transition has been described as 'the most dramatic socio-economic, cultural, and geopolitical change France had experienced since the Revolution' (Bousquet & Pessin, 2003, p. 46).

However, all was not smooth, especially with the ongoing conflict in its former colonies in South East Asia and Africa. Political turmoil over the Algerian fight for independence brought down the Fourth Republic in 1958. This was followed by the election of Charles de Gaulle as President, with a promise to restore order. At the same time, there was concern about the growing influence of American consumer culture, leading to the introduction of import quotas on American films and a greater promotion of 'Frenchness' throughout the nation (Hewitt, 2003). There were moves to foster greater European unity with the establishment of the European Economic Community in 1957. However, with the growing prosperity, there was a certain resistance to De Gaulle's authoritarian rule, which subsequently burst forth in the 1968 riots.

The artistic and cultural heritage of France was re-asserted. Artists and literary figures had attained great prominence in the public domain. These included Jean-Paul Sartre and Albert Camus, who tackled existentialist issues in their writings, reflecting the post-war trauma and the mighty changes that followed in French society. These and other works set out an agenda which, for many, reflected the disorientation they felt after surviving the horrors of the war. However, with the rise of consumerism in the 1960s, these ideas began to decline (Hewitt, 2003).

5.2.1 *Santé et maladie: ses images et ses publics*

It was within this historic context that Claudine Herzlich began her study of the social representations of health and illness in early 1960s France. A report of her findings was published in 1969 and an English translation followed four years later (Herzlich, 1973). This study remains the benchmark against which more recent studies can be compared. It is valued for its originality in terms of theory and methods, introducing social representation theory to the English-speaking world, as well as championing qualitative methods at a time when quantitative methods were dominant within social psychology.

Her research involved non-directive interviews with a sample of 80 French adults who were employed in professional and middle-class occupations. These participants were chosen 'because of the active role which it seemed reasonable to attribute to them in the genesis, transformation and renewal of ideologies in our society' (p. 13). Of the total sample of 80 participants, most were residents of Paris, but 12 were drawn from a small village in Normandy. The inclusion of this sub-sample was considered a 'limited attempt to include a style of life variable, which may reasonably be supposed to be important in matters of health and illness' (p. 14). The sample was divided 'more or less equally' (p. 13) in terms of age (25–40 vs. more than 40 years) and sex. Of note, 24% of her sample were ill at the time of the study, 13% had previously been seriously ill, and 20% had had an accident. Twenty of the original participants were re-interviewed and asked to comment on a transcription of their initial interview.

The interview was structured around a series of themes, the order and wording of which varied. The interview started with the request: 'I would like you to speak about health and illness, about your experience of them, and about what it represents for you' (p. 14). Herzlich emphasized that she wanted to avoid discussion of medical knowledge but rather to encourage discussion on how people felt about health and illness.

Later, reflecting on this research, Herzlich (2018) recalled that when she had completed the interviews, she was unsure how to interpret them and searched for a theoretical framework. It was then that she came across the work of Eliot Freidson, an American sociologist who had explored the social understanding of health and illness. According to Freidson (1961–1962), the sick person has a different view of illness from that of the physician, which can often draw them into conflict. Herzlich was keen to expand upon the layperson's view of health and illness.

The transcripts were subjected to a form of content analysis. Initially, this was inductive, but she also drew upon the work of the French philosopher and physician Canguilheim ([1943]1972), whose work focused on the meaning of normal and abnormal in medicine. In addition, she drew on the work of her supervisor Stoetzel (1960), who aimed to bring together ideas from sociology and psychology in the creation of social psychology. This reaching out to other disciplines illustrates the interdisciplinary nature of research on social representations.

Her unit of analysis for the interviews was a case or an individual participant, such that she was able to look within an individual interview and identify relationships between elements. For this reason, her analysis resulted in a more integrated approach to understanding social representations of health and illness, rather than a mere listing of themes.

Social representations of health: Herzlich wanted to explore 'the social representations of illness and health as realities *sui generis*, independent of medical models' (Herzlich, 2001, p. 193). She initially described three conceptions of health in her interviews with French adults. The first she termed *health-in-a-vacuum*. This was what her participants referred to as the absence of illness. She quoted one of her participants:

> Health is in short to live without noticing that time is passing; I think that if one day I wake up and I'm seventy, and I've lived like that, then I'll say that's good health ... in short, it will have been life without incidents (p. 56).

Besides this absence, some participants defined health in terms of a lack of awareness of the body. This definition of health had no psychological aspects but was simply the 'negation of illness'. Further, she described the relationship between health and illness as asymmetrical—'illness is the only point of reference, the only experience, the only incident' (p. 56).

The second conception was the *reserve of health*. This conception defined health as a social asset rather than a state' (p. 56). This asset had two aspects: on the one hand, physical robustness or strength, and on the other, potential for resistance to attacks, fatigue or illness. An example is the comment by one participant: 'I've always had a steady constitution, a reserve of robust health; I think I'm pretty resistant and not at all one of those with weak and precarious health' (p. 56).

This reserve, or 'capital asset', was not fixed but could vary over the lifespan depending upon circumstances. As another participant said: 'I see people as much as ten years younger than me who already have white hair because they have passed the whole of their lives shut up in offices or little rooms. Certainly, I attribute my capital health to the fact that I've lived more in the open air' (p. 57).

The participants often felt that childhood was a key period for developing a person's reserve of health. As one said:

> In a child, I think you have got to get them to build up their strength when they are young. Perhaps it's an odd kind of theory, but I think that what's acquired when you are a child is never lost ... it's always a good basis (p. 57).

This reserve of health also provided a defence against possible illness. Herzlich added that it is the 'substructure' of other types of health. It was something to build health upon. Furthermore, it allows a certain degree of personal control over health and illness. Here, one participant recalled from personal experience: 'When I was ill, many people would have been very much reduced by it ... I held out; I concluded that I owed it to my reserve of health' (p. 58).

The third conception of health was *equilibrium*. By this, it was meant a personal experience that all is well with yourself and your relationships. One participant summed up this experience: 'When I am enjoying good health, I feel well, there's a sense of equilibrium when I feel that everything is going well, and difficulties appear quite insignificant' (p. 58). This conception was sometimes termed 'real health'. It was the core aspect of health:

> There is not being ill ... but there is also real health, when the body functions like a well-oiled machine, without having to be looked after ... and there's also having sparkling eyes, a good color, to feel at ease when you meet up with friends, and not be at all on edge (p. 58).

The concept of equilibrium was central to the sense of health, but what exactly it was remained unclear. As Herzlich noted:

> Despite, or perhaps because of, the relative absence of precise meaning, a kind of agreement becomes established between discussants on the basis of repeated use of the same terms on the wide range of implicit meaning (p. 60).

She continued to list various themes that were mentioned by the participants and that she included in equilibrium. These included 'physical well-being, plenty of physical resources, absence of fatigue, psychological well-being, evenness of temper, freedom of movement, effectiveness in action, good relations with other people, as well as physical well-being' (p. 60). She concluded that this concept included 'personal, physical and social dimensions'.

The equilibrium conception of health implied 'an abundance, even a super-abundance of energy'. This abundance of energy could hold out the potential for use and abuse. The person can over-exert themselves because of this potential. It can also be regarded as a synonym for activity, 'a kind of activity at once unstrained and effective' (p. 61). One of the participants described it this way: 'I think equilibrium supposes a continuous state of activity... it is optimism, to want to do something, a kind of continuous dynamism' (p. 61).

This equilibrium could overcome organic illness. Thus, a person who is ill has the potential for health. As another participant said:

> For me, there is no such thing as perfect health, it's much more a matter of being able to keep a balanced life ... to be slightly ill, for example to have a tendency to bronchitis isn't to be in bad health, nor even having mild attacks of asthma. I'm in good health when I am in equilibrium, when I feel capable of doing what I want (p. 61).

This type of health refers to something one either has or does not have. It is a feeling one has about their health. An example given: 'When I am enjoying good health, I feel well, there's a sense of equilibrium when I feel that everything is going well, and difficulties appear quite insignificant' (p. 58).The term equilibrium was one that was used frequently by the participants but was not clearly defined. It was a state of being that could be conveyed to others. Here, Herzlich makes a rare comparison with Moscovici's (1961) work on social representations of psychoanalysis, in which he discussed the term 'complex', which he argued has a twofold function: descriptive/informative and symbolic. While the former function can provide detail, the latter symbolic function allows the speaker to locate the term in the broader field of psychoanalysis without detailed understanding. The same could be said for equilibrium, which is placed within the broader field of health. Herzlich stressed the

Table 5.1 Social representations of health

	Health-in-a-vacuum	*Reserve of health*	*Equilibrium*
	Being	*Having*	*Doing*
Content	Absence of positive content	Robustness and strength Resistance to attacks	Physical well-being good humour Activity good relations with others
Relation to person	Impersonal fact All or nothing	Personal characteristic Measurable, variable and permanent Secondary awareness	Personal norm All or nothing Immediate awareness
Relation to health	–	Basis of equilibrium	Based on reserve of other forms
Relation to illness	Destroyed by illness	Resistance to illness	Assimilation of disorders

Source Herzlich (1973)

centrality of this process: '[it] is the key which opens the world of health, the symbol which transports us there' (p. 60).

Distinguished between these three different conceptions of health using the terms being, having, and doing (Table 5.1). In Herzlich's model, *being* is health in a vacuum, *having* is a reserve of health and *doing* is equilibrium.

Further, she argued that there are two underlying aspects of health. First, there is the organic, which is concerned with the body—a relative state defined in terms of the presence of illness and resistance to it. Second, there is the psychosocial or behavioural aspect, which is concerned with the relationship of the person to the environment. The interaction of these two aspects leads to equilibrium or true health.

Social representations of illness: Herzlich contrasted the social representations of illness with those of health. Illness was defined in terms of the relationship between the active individual and society. Herzlich identified three conceptions of illness. The first she termed *illness as destructive*. This conception was prominent among participants who felt that they were very active and socially engaged. For them, being reduced to inactivity was the essence of illness. There were two main features of this conception: the feeling that the loss of social role had been imposed and the feeling that inactivity results in the destruction of social ties and solitude. For these people, involvement in social life and a clear social role were central to their identity. Related to this was pride in self-sufficiency. To be dependent on other people was distressing. This social exclusion, inactivity, and dependency were perceived as the loss of life—a form of death. If this happens early in life, it can impair the person's ability to become fully healthy in later life. Herzlich gives an example of a man who had asthma since childhood, who recounted that 'potentials of energy within me were stifled by the fact that I was too spoilt when I was a kid, as a sick child …' (p. 109). However, such inactivity and social exclusion could also have benefits, such as increased sensitivity.

There were various ways to combat the destructive aspects of illness. One was to deny that certain afflictions were serious and, if possible, to carry on as if nothing was wrong. Related to this strategy was the avoidance of seeking medical attention and the concealment of receiving treatment. However, this was not always possible, and then the person becomes really ill. This is termed passivity, when the patient can no longer deny or challenge the illness but must accept it and the associated treatment. Here, the person becomes a patient who is separate from the self.

The second conception was *illness as a liberator,* which involved a lessening of social responsibilities. It was an opportunity to abandon onerous responsibilities and even to blot out everyday reality. For many, it was compared to a holiday. Herzlich defined two conceptions of illness as a liberator. The first was rest and release from social obligations, which was commonly associated with benign and limited illnesses. The second was more dramatic and confined to serious illness and even death. Released from social obligations, there were certain benefits: i) new intellectual activities, ii) opportunities for contemplation and solitude, and iii) privileges from others because of one's illness.

Within this representation of illness was the conception of health as being the social norm, which limited opportunities for self-fulfilment for the invalid. However, there were three opportunities for growth of the invalid personality: (i) liberation from social constraints, (ii) personal transformation, and (iii) development of the exceptional personality: 'The invalid grows in stature because he suffers and because he has an experience which others do not have' (p. 117).

The third conception was termed *illness as an occupation* that accepts that the illness is real and that the patient has to struggle against it. Freed from social responsibilities, the patient has the resources to fight the illness. This becomes the person's new occupation. There are two basic factors in this struggle: acceptance of the illness and power over the illness. The power is evidenced in the ability to endure the illness and the associated pain, learning to live with it. The power is also evident in the ability of the patient to participate in the treatment and potential cure of the illness. Here, it is important that the patient has an adequate reserve of health to combat the illness. Recovering from illness, the person emerges stronger. While in the case of acute illness, the person can aim at achieving a cure, in the case of chronic illness, the aim is more one of adjustment to a different form of life. In doing so, the ill person 'asserts the enduring nature of his belongingness to society' (p. 125). He (or she) is not content with the social restraints but aims to be as full a participant in society as possible.

The most important determining factor of illness is the way of life, which is a function of your position in society. Health is something a person possesses, offering resistance to external threats. It also acts as a reserve, enabling the person to adjust to life.

Individual and society: Herzlich went beyond the description of social representations of health and illness to develop an understanding of how these phenomena are positioned within the relationship between the individual and society. She argued that health and illness were conceived as 'the outcome of a struggle between the individual equals health and way of life equals disease' (p. 26). In this struggle, we have the opposition of an 'active' factor, the way of life, which, by its incursions, leads to disease, and a 'passive' type (passive being synonymous with resistance), representing the perfect health of the individual (or the perfectly healthy individual). She summarized her model as the tension between the individual and society.

Way of life was positioned as the central dynamic linking health and illness, but what was this way of life? Herzlich summarized it as 'life in towns. In fact, it is life in Paris that its citizens without exception refer to' (p. 20). For example, one participant said: 'Paris is fatigue and nervous tension, with exhausting and rather unhealthy life'. Another added: 'The constant commotion isn't made to make people ordinary, they are difficult, nervous, tired; that's the truth about modern life' (pp. 20–21). One participant placed this way of life within a historical context:

> I have the impression that these diseases of today didn't exist in former times, just as the diseases of former times are no longer with us today. I feel we, well, not we but external circumstances and social conditions, create

> new sources of illness which, while still being called illnesses, take and more and more diverse and complicated forms (p. 22).

Herzlich connected this comment with its historical heritage. In particular, she referred to the contribution of the eighteenth-century French philosopher Jean-Jacques Rousseau (1712–1778), who had popularized the idea that people are naturally good but are corrupted by society.

Herzlich went on to describe how our understanding of health and illness is linked with our understanding of their genesis—a sociogenetic approach. Illness is due to the conflict between society, mediated by way of life, and the resistance of the individual with its 'reserve of health'. Health and illness can also be regarded as both a state and a conduct. As a state, it is something belonging to the individual, while as conduct, it involves the activity of the person.

Setting: As already mentioned, the 1960s was a period of intense social change in France. The Second World War created traumatic upheaval in French society—politically, socially, and psychologically. It was less than 20 years since the end of the war, which meant that those interviewed by Herzlich (25–40 years and 40+ years old) had lived through it and experienced the hardships and disruption caused by it. Many were children then, but assuming the average age was 40 years, the majority were young adults at the time and would have been able to recall its impact clearly. Herzlich was born in 1932 and so would have been a child during the war. Since then, she and her study participants had experienced the great reconstruction of French society.

The middle-class participants in Herzlich's study had lived through this dramatic social change, but they also felt ill at ease with the speed of this change. In their social representations of health, the participants in Herzlich's study were expressing unease at the rapid urbanization of society and the 'constant commotion', which they contrasted with the slower pace of rural life from which many of them would have come and with which they were familiar. This new 'way of life' was the main driver of ill-health. Farr (1977), commenting on the middle-class composition of the study sample, concluded that, based upon the study findings, 'one could with confidence invest in the marketing of Chambourcy or Loseley yogurts and other "natural" "health" foods to the middle-class denizens of Paris and London' (p. 501). But there was something more about the French participants' social representation of health.

Equilibrium was considered the core of 'real health'. The term was drawn from the interviews. In France, at that time, the term also reflected the growing political equilibrium in Europe with the formation of the European Economic Community. Moscovici ([1976] 2008) also discussed equilibrium in his analysis of the workings of social representations. 'The principle of equilibrium or cognitive consistency assumes that individuals avoid states of cognitive tension and that they prefer states in which cognitions and perceptions are all in agreement' (pp. 178–181). Here, he is referring to Heider's (1946) balance theory, which Heider developed as part of his 'naïve psychology'.

Equilibrium could be considered at different levels (cf. Doise, 1986). At the individual level, it is concerned with how one feels within oneself. It could be considered at the interpersonal level, which is concerned with relationships with others. It could also be considered at the societal level, where it is concerned with broader societal relations. At the societal level, equilibrium is less likely a term that would be applied to French society today. A qualitative study of young people conducted in the early 2010s found that many of them expressed pessimism about their future prospects and societal (dis)integration. They were anxious about their control over entry to the labour market and their life opportunities (Mary, 2014). Many felt very uneasy about the future. A European survey of people aged 16–29 years found that only 4% of French respondents agreed with the statement, 'Society's future looks bright' (Galland, 2008). After being appointed Prime Minister of France in 2024, Michel Barnier said that his first task would be to 'respond as best we can to the challenges, the anger, the feeling of abandonment and injustice that is too prevalent in our cities, on our estates, and in the countryside' (Chrisafis, 2024).

The decline in the importance of balance or equilibrium was evident in a study conducted in the 2010s on social representations of health in modern France (Aim et al., 2018). The researchers used Abric's structural model as their analytic framework, which was designed to identify the core and peripheral elements of social representations. For this, they employed a lexical study design in which 120 adults were asked to produce four words that they spontaneously associated with 'health'. Participants were then asked to rank these four words in order of importance and to produce a phrase to contextualize each word.

Table 5.2 Frequency and importance of health terms

Frequency	*Importance*	
	High	*Low*
High	Well-being Illness Doctor Sport Medication	Hospital
Low	Balance Good, good shape Life, happiness Care, medical Healthy lifestyle Prevention, good mood	Diet Longevity Freedom Cancer

Source Aim et al. (2018)

The words were then subjected to a lexicographical analysis to see in what way the words clustered together in terms of frequency and perceived importance. Table 5.2 summarizes the frequency of the different terms and their importance for the participants. Although balance was rated as important, it was not mentioned frequently. Well-being was considered more important.

In subsequent work, Herzlich further expanded her discussion of the socio-historical locatedness of health and illness. In their historical study of changing representations of illness, Herzlich and Pierret (1984) noted how memory of previous negative experiences pervaded understandings of illness. As they remarked: 'The memory of the terrors of the past remained astonishingly vivid'. Or, as Sulivan (2000), the French theologian, remarked: 'You never live in the present. The present only leaves us with an image of the past which we relive painfully' (p. 23). The characterization of illness as liberation might have been a reflection of the experience of those participants in Herzlich's study who were ill or who had had an illness. Marcel Proust, who suffered from severe asthma, wrote of the benefits of illness—*sur le bon usages des mauvaises santés* (Proust, [1902]2022). This is not an experience that was apparent in subsequent studies of social representations of illness among healthy adults.

The terms that Herzlich used also have historical precedents. She not only drew upon Freidson's sociological ideas of social action but also

Sartre's existentialism. In his classic *Being and Nothingness*, Sartre ([1943] 2020) differentiated between three relations to an object that can be projected in desiring: *being*, *doing* and *having*. These are the terms Herzlich used to describe the different illness experiences. As Moscovici emphasized, ideas are rooted in the intellectual climate of the time, even when this is not recognized (Moscovici, 1998, p. 413). In addition, while being and having can be considered as part of the process of objectification, doing is the process of anchoring. It is through doing that the person maintains social activity and equilibrium within themselves and with others.

Similarly, in her descriptions of social representations of illness, Herzlich used the terms destruction, occupation and liberation (*la maladie destructice, la maladie-métier, la maladie-libératrice*), which have a historical resonance. In France, the war-time experience has been described in terms of *l'occupation, collaboration and resistance* (Davies, 2001; Porch, 2024). There is a similarity in the terms used by Herzlich to characterize illness with those used to describe wartime experience. This is especially the case in the English version, which translates *métier* as occupation. Although the terms may have different meanings, there is an echo between the two experiences. All three experiences reflect different forms of doing, of engaging with the social world.

Qualitative interviews were the primary source of data in Herzlich's research. At that time, quantitative and experimental research were dominant in American and British social psychology, where the aim was to create a natural science. In France, historically, the education system throughout the twentieth century balanced the humanities with the sciences. Today, the study of literature and the arts remains important in French lycées and in French political life. Herzlich included extensive extracts from a sample of the interviews in the Appendix to the study. Review of these reveal the narrative content of the interviews with the participants detailing examples of health and illness from their everyday lives (László, 1997). The three-fold characterization of illness could also be considered a reflection of the dominant narrative structures suggested by Gergen and Gergen (1973), viz., liberation - progresssive, destruction - regressive, and occupation - stable (Murray, 2002).

Farr (1977) suggested that the use of interviews encouraged a certain attributional bias in the views expressed by the participants. According to Heider's (1958) attribution theory, people attribute causes to events they encounter. There is a tendency to attribute the cause of success to the self and the cause of failure to the environment. In Herzlich's study, the participants attributed the source of health to the person and that of illness to the environment or the modern way of life. Herzlich (1993) responded that while Farr's suggestion was innovative, it did not annul the modern representation of illness as being due to real or symbolic external forces. Her identification of these external forces was not modern but was also apparent in historical sources. She referred to *la vision rousseauiste*, the view of Jean-Jacques Rousseau (1712–1778), according to whom people were good before the development of civilization. For example, he wrote in *A Dissertation on the Origin and Foundation of the Inequality of Mankind and Is It Authorized by Natural Law?* (1754):

> Excesses of every kind, immoderate transports of every passion, fatigue, mental exhaustion, the innumerable pains and anxieties inseparable from every condition of life, by which the mind of man is incessantly tormented; these are too fatal proofs that the greater part of our ills are of our own making, and that we might have avoided them nearly all by adhering to that simple, uniform, and solitary manner of life that nature prescribed (in Herzlich, 1973, p. 31).

This identification of illness as being 'of our own making', of the person as being responsible for ill-health, remains. We are naturally healthy, but it is the nature of our society that leads us to ill-health. However, this is not straightforward as subsequent studies by Blaxter (1990) and other illustrate (see below).

5.2.2 *Personal and Social Norms in the 1970s*

Between 1971 and 1974, a related study was conducted by d'Houtaud and Field (1984) in Nancy, a historic city in the north-east of France. After the upheavals of the 1960s, France had settled somewhat with the election of the conservative George Pompidou as President in 1970. This was a period of continued modernization of the economy, a decline in the influence of the Communist Party and the rise of identity politics (Chabal, 2000).

A written questionnaire was administered to 4000 residents who attended for a health examination in the city. Unlike Herzlich's study, the study sample included a large proportion of manual workers. The questionnaire included an open-ended question requesting a definition of health. The responses were content-analysed into 41 themes, which were,

Table 5.3 Classifications of the ten groupings of themes of health

	Series A	*Series B*
	Predominance of the 'I', of internalization, of personal norms	Predominance of the 'one', of externalization, of social norms
1. Objective criteria	Hedonistic use of life	Value of health
2. Subjective criteria	Reference to the body	Psychological well-being
3. Means	Equilibrium	Hygiene, Prevention
4. Objectives	Vitality	Absence of sickness Physical aptitudes

Adapted from d'Houtaud and Field (1984)

in turn, reduced to ten categories classified by socio-economic status. The most common category among the higher and middle-class respondents was *hedonistic use of life*, *equilibrium*, *reference to the body* and *vitality*, while among the more manual workers, the most common categories were *prevention*, *physical aptitudes* and *absence of sickness*.

A bipolar structure was then proposed to organize these ten categories. This is presented in Table 5.3. Series A was the dominant approach among the higher and middle socio-economic groupings. It focused on the 'I' and the hedonistic use of life. Series B was dominant among the manual workers and focused on the value of health. In Series A, the 'I', 'internalization' and personal norms predominated, while in Series B, the 'one', 'externalization' and social norms predominated. This would suggest that, for the higher and middle classes, the realization of the self predominates, while for the manual workers, there is a more socialized conception of self.

The authors concluded that this bipolar representation of health reflected the orientation to self or to society:

> Is this not a verification that the representation of health is as much a model of behaviour meant to be applied to social reality as a cognitive reflection of the values and of the knowledge current in society? Is this not as much as much the concrete reaction of the individual who integrates himself more with his social environment, or of the one who chooses to dominate it for his advantage, as it is communication among the members of a community? Is it

not a faithful witness of the conflicts that oppose social partners and their manner of perceiving their reciprocal interest? (p. 53).

Another point was concern with the body. For the higher and middle classes, the body was for the enjoyment of life, while for the manual workers, it was for the service of society during work. Together, these studies illustrated the social locatedness of social representations of health and illness in time and place. This was apparent in studies conducted in other locations.

5.3 Adults in 1980s Britain and Ireland

In the previous chapter, we discussed the social and political changes happening in Britain in the 1980s. Following the so-called *Winter of Discontent* throughout Britain, which witnessed sustained industrial strife, Margaret Thatcher was elected Prime Minister in 1979 as the head of a Conservative government that was to rule for the following 14 years. This was a period of economic retrenchment, with major cuts to social services, the privatization of nationalized industries and the sell-off of council houses. The government strongly promoted a policy of individual responsibility, epitomized in the advice of Norman Tebbit, the Junior Minister, to millions of unemployed workers to 'get on your bike' and seek work. It was also the period that saw the rise of punk music, which reflected a broader cultural shift. It emphasized a do–it-yourself philosophy, with the associated belief in autonomous social and political action against the constraints of the corporate elites. As the punk rocker Joey Ramone advised at that time: 'Play before you get good, because by the time you get good, you're too old to play'. It was during this period that several studies of social representations of health and illness were conducted in different regions of Britain and Ireland.

5.3.1 *Middle Englanders*

In the late 1980s, a study was conducted in England by Stainton-Rogers (1991). Stainton-Rogers was a social psychologist based at the Open University in Britain who had been engaged in sustained discussions about the nature of social psychology and alternative research methods (Curt, 1994). Her study adopted a Q-sort methodology, which involves a combination of qualitative and quantitative techniques. It begins by using in-depth interviews to solicit details of people's views about a particular phenomenon. The researchers then extract from the interview transcripts the key statements that convey their views. The study participants are then asked to arrange these statements in a so-called Q-grid. The statements are subsequently reduced through a process of factor analysis to certain primary accounts of the phenomenon.

This approach was developed in the 1930s by William Stephenson while working in London with the psychometricians Charles Spearman and Cyril Burt, but it was largely forgotten when he moved to the United States. It was reinvigorated in the 1990s by Rex and Wendy Stainton-Rogers and, since then, has attracted the interest of some qualitative researchers as a means of identifying patterns of human subjectivity. Its focus has been on clarifying 'the subjective dimension of any issue towards which *different points-of-view* can be expressed' (Stenner et al., 2008, p. 215).

Using this approach, Stainton-Rogers began her study by talking with six men and seven women in England about health and illness. This small sample included academics, health professionals, and some from other middle-class and working-class occupations. She conducted detailed semi-structured interviews with these people and extracted over 650 statements about health and illness. After excluding those concerned with social policy and funding issues, she reduced this number to 506 statements that were focused on explanations of health and illness. After a series of statistical exercises designed to reduce this number to a core grouping of 80 statements, she administered these to a sample of 70 participants who were asked to complete a series of Q-sort grids. This final sample of participants included health professionals and individuals from a range of other occupations. The 70 participants' completed Q-sort response grids were then subjected to factor analysis, from which she extracted seven primary accounts. These were named: *cultural critique, willpower, health promotion, body as machine, inequality of access, body under siege* and *robust individualism.*

She then conducted a second study linking health control items with the multi-dimensional health locus of control scale (Wallston et al., 1978). This time, the Q-sort included items concerned with health control. The participants in this study were drawn from a more diverse population and included more individuals from a working-class background compared with the previous study. Factor analysis of the 83 grids completed identified six primary accounts: *willpower, body as machine, body under siege, cultural critique, God's power* and *robust individualism.*

Taking these two studies together, Stainton-Rogers developed eight main accounts of health and illness:

1. Body as machine: operating with the modernist view of science.
2. Body under siege: the individual is under threat from germs and diseases.
3. Inequality of access: benefits of modern medicine are unfairly distributed.
4. Cultural critique: emphasis on exploitation and oppression.
5. Health promotion: collective and personal responsibility for health.
6. Robust individualism: individual's right to a satisfying life.
7. God's power: spiritual well-being and God's care.
8. Willpower: individual in control.

Although people could draw upon these different accounts, there was also a preference for certain accounts among different groups. Thus, the political radicals would prefer the cultural critique account, which involved a broader critique of the role of science and medicine. The *God's power* account was preferred by those with strong religious convictions.

In conclusion, Stainton-Rogers suggested that 'people have access to and utilize a range of alternative accounts to "make sense of" health and illness' (p. 226). She used the ecological term 'sympatricity' to describe this process of competing accounts. Sympatric accounting is 'perhaps more broadly approachable as a process of "making sense" of a difficult topic by reference to a variety of texts of different kinds' (p. 227). Furthermore, she suggested a narrative means of integrating these different texts through a process of storytelling. 'A theory of explanation based upon a notion of account sympatricity is thus one which portrays people as storymakers who weave a narrative in and out of different "texts"' (p. 228).

Taken together, this integrative framework is a sort of narrative version of cognitive polyphasia. It is a means of selecting from a virtual library of explanations the one most appropriate. Our understanding of health and illness is variable, as 'we never read texts in literal isolation, but always against the backcloth of all the other texts which we are consulting' (Stainton Rogers, 1991, p. 227). Indeed, Moscovici remarked, 'We are born into a large library in which we find all kinds of knowledge, of idioms, of norms and so on' (Moscovici & Marková, 1998, p. 382). Other studies suggest that the process of selecting and connecting resources from such a library is not simply rational but one filled with emotions, historical experience and the contemporary context.

5.3.2 *Women in Scotland*

In the early 1980s, a study that adopted a complementary approach to that of Herzlich was conducted by Mildred Blaxter. Blaxter was a British sociologist who had worked with Rory Williams in Aberdeen (see Chap. 7). She reviewed the evidence from the National Health and Lifestyle Survey, which was conducted in the late 1980s in Britain (Blaxter, 1990). This survey found that behavioural factors, such as poor diet and lack of exercise, were overwhelmingly identified as the cause of specific diseases and ill-health in general. Health was also defined in terms of behaviour as epitomized in this question and answer: 'Why do you call [a chosen person] healthy? I call her healthy because she goes jogging and she doesn't drink alcohol'. Conversely, environmental factors were mentioned less frequently. It seemed that the government's public policy—'you are responsible for your health'—had been widely accepted. Those with higher incomes were more likely to refer to environmental and structural factors. This tendency of working-class people to attribute the cause of ill-health to behaviours was similar to some earlier, smaller studies (Blaxter, 1993; Pill & Stott, 1985).

To explore this apparent conundrum, Blaxter conducted biographical interviews with a sample of 47 Scottish working-class women who were aged around 50 years (Blaxter & Patterson, 1982). This study found that the women balanced an awareness of their difficult childhood and circumstances with accepting responsibility for their current behavioural choices. Although they presented their childhood as being difficult, it was also described as in a way 'healthier' in the sense of 'good food, fresh air and sensible living' (p. 129). These healthy and tough childhoods provided them with a 'reserve of good health' such that they were more able to combat current adversity.

These women were aware of the link between social deprivation in their early years, but this conflicted with accounts of childhood rural life as healthy, with lots of fresh air and simple, good food. For example, one woman said:

> We were a healthy family. The country people are more healthy than the town people. They have more fresh air, there's not so much traffic, factories, things like that. And we lived off the land, more or less, there wasn't so much tinned stuff and things like that ... Their whole way of life has a lot to do wi' it (p. 130).

It was suggested that these women felt that these healthy childhoods had provided them with a certain 'reserve of good health, better to withstand the attacks that later life circumstances might make' (p. 130).

As with Herzlich (1973), Blaxter attempted to explore the linkages within the various biographical accounts. Most prominent was the concern with life events. These were especially associated with the female role and included childbearing, care of elderly relatives, menopause, widowhood and child death. The second feature of the accounts was 'the strain to connect, to present a health history as a chain of cause and effect' (p. 137). This strain to connect was reflected in the importance of family history, which was, in some ways, 'a desire to give meaning to their lives' (p. 138).

At the core of these biographical accounts was a desire to present a moral identity. The women were struggling in their everyday social interactions to maintain their sense of moral integrity. While they might have had, and still have, difficult circumstances, they were not succumbing to them but struggling to maintain their own health and that of their children. Despite their adverse current circumstances, they felt that they could not be ill because of their maternal responsibilities. As one mother said:

> When they were young, if I was ill, I couldn't afford to be ill and that was all there was to it. Because he [husband] was at sea and there was naebody. There wasn't anyone to watch the kids. If I was ill I still had to get up and work, you know – you couldn't be ill (p. 131).

It was not that the women were neglecting the importance of social conditions, but rather they were active social beings whose worth depended upon their ability to challenge these conditions. It was considered wrong, or even bad, to lie down when illness was encountered. As one woman said:

> 'I never lie down to illness - I've gotten up in the morning wi' a migraine and gone to work. Nearly killed me, but I've gone... I'd rather be out in company, you know, an' you're busy' (p. 139).

Work was an integral part of their accounts. Blaxter suggested that this was part of the Protestant work ethic which pervaded their society and which we consider in Chap. 7. The important point was the reluctance of these working class women to attribute the cause of ill-health to the environment. Central to their identity was the acceptance of responsibility for their health.

5.3.3 *Women in 1980s Northern Ireland*

In the late 1980s, Northern Ireland was a society slowly emerging from two decades of civil strife. The so-called Troubles were rooted in the sectarian divisions in the north of Ireland, which had existed for several hundred years and were entrenched by the partition of the island of Ireland in 1920. Since then, there had been periodic episodes of sectarian violence, often followed by the repression of the Catholic/Nationalist minority by the Protestant/Unionist government. During the 1960s, there were increasing demands for greater civil rights and equal opportunities for Catholics. This was opposed by the Unionist majority, leading to increasing social conflict. In the 1970s, there were over 2000 conflict-related deaths and thousands more non-fatal injuries in a population of 1.5 million.[1] Various attempts were made to bring about some political settlement, which led to a reduction in deaths, but there continued to be upsurges in violence throughout the 1980s.

In the late 1980s, a study of social representations of health and illness among working-class women in the city of Derry was conducted (Murray & McMillan, 1988). Derry is a city of about 100,000 people, which had been at the centre of political violence for almost 20 years. It was where the infamous Bloody Sunday massacre occurred in 1972, in which 13 innocent civilians were killed by the British Army. In 1982, a bomb exploded in a bar outside the city, killing eleven soldiers and six civilians. In the later 1980s, there was a lull in the killings, but a dreadful event occurred in 1987 when one student and two policemen were killed on the university campus in the city where the research team was based. In addition, Derry has experienced decades of both political and social discrimination. The unemployment rates and measures of disadvantage were higher here than in other areas of Northern Ireland. However, there remained an intense pride in the place despite the deprivation. This is portrayed in the lyrics of the popular song *The Town I Loved So Well* (1973) by the local songwriter Phil Coulter: 'And when times got rough there was just about enough/But they saw it through without complaining/For deep inside was a burning pride/For the town I loved so well'. The various churches remained a very influential cultural force, with both the Catholic and Protestant churches preaching strong conservative moral values. Church attendance remained very high, especially among Catholics.

[1] The population of the UK was around 55 million at that time such that an equivalent UK-wide death toll would have been around 70,000.

It was within this social and political context that the study was conducted. The aim was to explore how the social representations of health were entwined with notions of the participants' everyday lives. The study involved interviews and focus groups with a total sample of 37 women aged between 30 and 40 years, who came from a small working-class, mainly Catholic area near the centre of the city. Of these women, most of whom were young mothers, 19 were interviewed individually, and the remaining 18 participated in group discussions. The interviews/discussions were semi-structured and were conducted by one of the researchers, a middle-aged woman from a nearby area who was familiar with many of the local challenges. In the interviews, she introduced a variety of themes and, through interchange, encouraged the women to provide a detailed account of their views on health, illness and the health service. The interviews/discussions were all tape-recorded and then subsequently transcribed and reviewed. The analysis was generally inductive but was informed by the work of Herzlich. Particular attention was given to how the women perceived gender and social class differences in health experiences.

Social representations of health: When asked to describe health, the majority of women commented that it was something they had never really thought about before. Although they stated that they found it difficult to describe health, nevertheless, they provided a range of descriptive terms. There were three primary definitions of health similar to those identified by Herzlich, and a fourth that emphasized family health (Table 5.4).

Health as activity was concerned with the ability to perform everyday activities. For example, one woman said: 'You know when you're healthy enough ... able to go about your work and housework and everything

Table 5.4 Social representations of health in Derry

	Content	*Maintenance*
Activity	Able to do usual activities	Healthy behaviours
Personal	Feeling good	Nothing
Family	Healthy children	Childcare
Absence	Not illness	–

Source Murray and McMillan (1988)

like that ... that's what I call health, y'know'. The importance of health was the ability to go about their day-to-day lives without hindrance, e.g., 'You have to be healthy to get about every day, because if you're not healthy every day is a sort of chore to you really, you know'. This dimension was similar to Herzlich's equilibrium dimension, which is concerned with doing something.

This activity definition of health was matched with a behavioural definition of health maintenance. This included activities such as exercise, but particularly diet. For example, one woman said:

> Now even the children, they don't know the taste of butter any more. They really don't because I don't buy it. Again, wholemeal bread and skimmed milk, that's an accepted thing now with myself and all of them. All my family, brothers and sisters, all do the same, you know, taking bran and trying not to fry too much ... and chips, now at the most would be once a week ... maybe on a Saturday as a treat. I would encourage them to eat more fruit ... so it's something. It's as best as I know how anyway to try and keep them healthy.

The *health as a personal* dimension included references to general well-being or feeling good within yourself. This included references to being fit, e.g., 'I think it's how fit you feel'; 'Health is probably fitness of the body'. However, this was different from the fitness described by the young people in the previous chapter. One woman clarified the distinction between health and physical fitness:

> I think people get health and physical fitness confused. You know they think physical fitness ... you know, out training, out jogging, or out walking ... it's just pure health ... but not being sick, it's two different things.

This dimension was more concerned with the state of body and mind. For example: 'Feeling good, looking good, being happy' and 'Fitness ... I don't really know. I would say your ability to be able to manage your life'. Health was something you either did or did not have: 'I mean it's very important because if you haven't got your health, I mean you've nothing. Even if you had all the money in the world it wouldn't do you any good if you haven't got your health'. This is similar to Herzlich's Reserve of Health dimension. You didn't have to do anything extra, but you had it within yourself to handle any challenges.

A third dimension was *health and the family*. Health was something the women took more or less for granted unless they or some member of their family became ill, e.g.,

> To me as a mother ... not just my health but the family too, because when you have a family, it's very important that they're healthy too. Because I would find that if the children are sick or my husband would be ill, it does affect me. Maybe not physically but mentally ... if I would be worried about them, you know.

The family was of central importance to these women. They felt that the mother had to be healthy so as to look after the home and her children. As one woman said: 'Health is very important if you're rearing a family, for if you're not healthy, you're going to take it out on them... y'know. You can't do for them what you should be doing.'

This emphasis on the importance of motherhood was a reflection of the central role of family responsibility for these women. Health was anchored in motherhood, and being a good mother was its moral component.

Absence of illness was the fourth definition of health. This definition did not provide any details of health but rather defined it as the absence of illness. It was the 'being' definition of health, which Herzlich described as health-in-a-vacuum.

It was felt by many of the women that their greater responsibility for children and the family meant that they were more prone to illness than men. The main explanation for this was the difference in the family/work roles of men and women, e.g.,

> Women have a harder life than men, I always think. Women have to watch children, and with cooking and cleaning. They say it must be great staying in the house all day, but I would rather be out working.

Women's reproductive role was also perceived as a reason for their poorer health. Other reasons given were that men play sports, go jogging and participate in physical activities more than women. A small number of women also suggested that men were less inclined to worry than women—worry being perceived as a cause of illness.

Over half of the women who provided details believed that people from middle-class backgrounds were healthier. Two explanations were given for this. Firstly, the women referred to the better diet of middle-class people.

Usually, this was considered to be due to their greater spending power. The second major explanation given by the women for the better health of middle-class people was that they generally had less stressful lives, e.g.,

> They don't feel the pressures of unemployment or a man being at home and feeling that he's not providing for his family ... I think that contributes to stress and anxiety and maybe ... not breakups, but certainly alcohol abuse.

It was also suggested that the middle classes could afford to have private medical treatment and, therefore, not have to remain on a waiting list for a long time.

Social representations of illness: A variety of descriptions of illness were given. These were largely concerned with different forms of disruption to the women's lives. They were organized into three categories, with an additional category that simply defined it as the absence of health.

Illness as social disruption defined illness in relation to the restrictions it places on everyday activities:

> I would consider illness something that affected a person's life on the whole as opposed to the odd ache or having some minor thing that you can still carry on with normal life ... Anything that would prevent you leading a normal life I suppose would be considered illness.

Illness as personal disruption had two components: physical and psychological. The physical component described illness in terms of something that affected some part of the body: 'You know there's something wrong ... aches, pains and whatever that you never had before'. The psychological component included references to mental illness when defining illness: 'Nervous illness ... that would be worries, depression, crying when you're on your own. I think that's the worst'.

Illness as family disruption is described in terms of its consequences for the family if they themselves or other members of the family are ill:

> Well, if there's illness in the family it affects everybody in the family. I mean if somebody's sick and they're in hospital, you're running to the hospital, you're worried about them, and it can affect the people who aren't sick more even than the person that actually is, after a length of time.

Illness, as absence, was simply the absence of health, e.g., 'It's a state of not being healthy'.

The women identified a wide range of causes of illness. These causes were initially broadly classified as personal (i.e., belonging to the individual) or impersonal. In addition, they were classified as controllable or not controllable (cf. Wallston & Wallston, 1978). The most frequently cited causes of illness were classified as *personal/controllable.* This included poor personal care, not looking after oneself properly by, for example, not eating proper food, not wearing warm clothes or not having health check-ups:

> I think maybe in some cases people maybe wouldn't look after themselves ... maybe in eating or just generally. Maybe too lazy to see about getting a check-up or things like that. I think maybe very six months or every year people should really go and get a good check-up. That could prevent illness, too.

A related category was poor diet, which was mentioned frequently. Smoking or drinking alcohol to excess were also regarded as potential causes of illness.

The second dimension was labelled *personal/uncontrollable* and included references to heredity and physical constitution. For example,

> Well, I think everybody starts out with a different set of equipment ... their bodies ... and some people are just more prone because maybe their parents before them were.

The *impersonal/uncontrollable* factors included viruses, food additives, nuclear waste and luck or chance. Although it could be suggested that the first three are controllable in the sense that certain preventive or protective behaviours could reduce their impact, they have all been classified as uncontrollable since they were often mentioned together. The women who referred to these factors tended to consider them part of contemporary civilization:

> I think it's just this day and age has a lot to do with it. There's a lot of canned stuff. Really, years ago they grew a lot of stuff, didn't they? And fresh. It's not that there isn't plenty of that at the minute but I think everybody is inclined to turn to the can opener too, aren't they, you know. It's a lot handier.

Some women believed that getting ill was just a matter of luck or chance. One woman said: 'Well, anybody can get an illness. I mean it just strikes out of the blue, you know.' Another added: 'How can you stop picking up disease. I mean there are some things that you just can't control.'

The women, however, tended not to attribute illness to a singular cause. In addition, several made the distinction between common illnesses such as flu, measles and so forth, and more serious illnesses such as cancer, attributing different causes to each:

> I honestly don't know why people become ill ... maybe not looking after themselves ... everyday illnesses I'm talking about, you know, like colds and flus and things like that. Maybe not giving their bodies enough vitamins. Not eating the proper sort of foods that they should eat. This is for colds and flus. I'm not talking about cancer or anything like that.

The general tenor of the views expressed was that the more common illnesses could be prevented to some degree by taking proper care of oneself, but this was less the case with the more serious illnesses, especially cancer.

Gender, class and health: These social representations of health and illness were intertwined with their representations of gender and social class. While Herzlich considered health representations among middle-class men and women, this study considered the particular processes involved in more working-class women in a society that had historically experienced social deprivation and political oppression.

For these women, a central part of their social representation of health was in terms of their family. Health meant a healthy family, and they worked to achieve this by caring for their children and promoting healthy lifestyles. As in Blaxter's (1993) study, the emphasis was on their moral standing as good mothers. They worked to not only maintain their own health but also that of their family. While the whole family may have experienced forms of social disadvantage, their discussion of these broader issues was confined to their reference to men. For these women, their lives were centred on home-life and their family. Broader social issues were more the concern of men. Health was vitally important to these women, especially in their role as mothers.

Conversely, the women viewed illness in terms of disruption to their everyday routines. Once again, the family was central. A wide range of factors were identified as causing illness. The most popular were personal and controllable factors, such as personal care and dietary control, suggesting that the women held themselves responsible for ill-health. However, in these cases, the ill-health was more of a minor type. More serious illnesses, such as cancer, were deemed to be outside of their control. Women were felt to be more prone to illness due largely to their reproductive role and their role in society. Most of the women thought that illness was not related to social class. While the disruptive side of illness was emphasized it was combined with a desire to return to health—illness as an occupation in Herzlich's terms. They worked hard to maintain good health in their family by promoting a healthy lifestyle. If they became ill, they had no desire to simply accept that illness. Rather, they worked to return to full health so that they could look after their children. There was no reference to illness as a liberator; it was always described in negative terms.

The underlying process in these social representations of health and illness was the struggle to be a good mother (cf. Hale et al., 2017). Motherhood was central to their social identity. Being a good mother meant keeping both self and children healthy and recovering quickly from illness. These working-class women strove to be good mothers, which meant caring for their children and promoting good health. The centrality of their identity as mothers was reflectd in their social representations of health and illness.

Derry was a city that had experienced sustained civil conflict over the previous generation and religious discrimination. Despite this, there was no reference to the broader political context or to religious factors. This might reflect a certain secularization of society or, alternatively, a certain muting of references to religion or politics in their accounts (Deschamps & Guimelli, 2002). Although questions on these topics were not included, there was possibly a hidden agenda. The women were from a mainly Catholic district, talking to an authority, and so were reluctant to discuss religion or politics. As the Irish poet Seamus Heaney wrote: 'Northern reticence, the tight gag of place/And times: yes, yes. Of the 'wee six' I sing/Where to be saved you only must save face/And whatever you say, you say nothing' (Heaney, 1975). Similarly, Guareschi and Jovchelovitch (2004) defined the law of silence as the strategy communities use to protect themselves from outsiders. By only revealing certain information, they deny access to the outsider.

5.4 Chinese Adults in 1990s England

Britain has increasingly become a multicultural society. Although this has accelerated over the past twenty years, there have been minority ethnic groups in the country for centuries. Britain has the oldest Chinese community in Europe, with the first immigrants from China arriving after the First Opium War in 1842. Since then, the size of the community has grown to around half a million, with the greatest density in London. In the 1990s, there were about 100,000 Chinese residents in London, most of whom were second or later generation, but many of whom could speak Chinese. The Chinese have a long-established medical tradition, but in England, they have been exposed to the Western medical tradition. This clash of medical traditions was explored in the late 1990s by Jovchelovitch and Gervais (1999).

Their study examined how Chinese residents talked about and performed health and illness. It used both individual interviews and focus groups, drawing on three different sources of data: interviews with six experts on the Chinese community, individual interviews with 12 adults and four focus groups with 24 adults. The analysis of the interview transcripts considered both the content and the underlying processes in the social representations. It was noted that 'the following representations did not occur as a fully articulated corpus of notions in the data. They emerged through story-telling and the description of everyday experiences and practices' (p. 251). They were often expressed in a 'patchy and fragmented form'. In addition, it was suggested that this was due, in part, to the fact that 'knowledge transmission in Chinese cultures relies more on rituals and on gestures than on explanation' (p. 251).

Two primary content themes were identified. The first theme emphasized the centrality of balance and harmony in representations of health and illness. This balance was both within the body and between the individual and the external social, natural and supernatural world. While this thme was similar to Herzlich's theme of equilibrium it was also clearly linked with the classic Chinese philosophy of Yin and Yang, which sees balance as intrinsic to the regulation of self and society. The study participants felt that vital energy circulates through the body and must be kept in balance. However, this belief expands to our relationship with the outer world, including harmony within the family and in our relationship with the world. Transmission of food habits plays an important part in ensuring that this knowledge is transferred to younger generations. Ch'I or Qi is this energy or life force which preserves harmony. As one expert said:

> You have to have balance. This is the Chinese point of view. This is why the country is called China. China is called the Middle Kingdom. We believe we're in the middle of the world, of the Earth. Everything must be nicely balanced. So, for example, if you have dry lips, blisters, or ulcers, you must be hot. In order to balance that, then you must take something, not necessarily medicine but soups and other remedies which have the cold properties in order to balance it (p. 253).

Illness was the symptomatic manifestation of energetic disequilibrium or insufficiency. It was caused either by internal or external factors.

Harmony within the family and respect for its hierarchy and fundamental values, the primacy of collective goals over individual needs and desires, obedience to authority and self-discipline all maintain the self in balance. It was from within 'an elaborate worldview embedded in ancient tradition that the Chinese community extracts the resources to construct a representational system about health and illness' (p. 253). However, although this was the dominant representational system, there were also elements of the Western system. It was this mixing of the Chinese with Western knowledge that was characteristic of the representations of health held by the Chinese community in London.

The second theme revolved around food rituals. In the interviews, it was apparent that the participants revealed their social representations of health through their discussion of their food rituals. Indeed, the discussion of food was central to their understanding of health. The priority given to food led the authors to conclude that 'together with language, food is probably the most important vehicle for the transmission of traditional health beliefs' in the Chinese community (p. 254).

Food was a means of objectifying understandings of health and a way of clearly providing a sense of Chinese identity. The use of food had an all-around value: it was a means of promoting health and treating illness. Furthermore, it was a means of transmitting health understandings across generations. The Chinese participants did not have any reflexive understanding of these health/food practices; rather, it was considered part of their culture. This was especially the case among older and more isolated members of the Chinese community.

Jovchelovitch and Gervais further argued that this ability to clearly verbalize the reasons for food or other health-related practices is a 'Western, modern phenomenon, deeply tied in with a particular kind of public sphere and democratic values' (p. 255). In Chinese and other more traditional cultures, it is through the observation of the practices of elderly and wise people that knowledge is transmitted. Harmony and the maintenance of harmony were central to their understanding of health and illness. This was an intrinsic part of Chinese culture but was concerned not just with internal harmony but also harmony with others.

This project demonstrates how social representations of health and illness are not just evident in accounts but also in the practices of the study participants. Furthermore, they are connected to the cultural identity of the participants. Maintaining a Chinese identity was important, and this was emphasized through food and health practices. The less acculturated members were also able to sustain both Western and Chinese health beliefs in a pragmatic manner. This did not threaten their Chinese identity, which was well established. Admittedly, the process of identity maintenance was an ongoing effort, continually challenged by the all-encompassing Western culture. Adopting Western foods and practices posed an existential threat to their identity. The nature of their social representations of health and illness revealed the tensions over identity experienced by younger members of the Chinese community and were often expressed through story-telling.

5.5 Adults in 2010s England

A recurrent theme in the study of social representations of health and illness has been the reference to the body. As already mentioned by Herzlich (2018), Moscovici had an early interest in researching social representations of the body. In her study of social representations of health (Herzlich, 1973), there was frequent reference to the body. A central aspect of 'health in a vacuum' was a lack of awareness of the body, e.g., 'the fact of not having a body, so to speak, it doesn't bother you in any way' (p. 56). The 'reserve of health' definition emphasized the organic-biological characteristics of the individual and health as a smoothly functioning body, e.g., 'when the body functions like a well-oiled machine, without having to be looked after' (p. 58).

Jodelet (1984) took up this interest in social representations of the body in a series of studies conducted in France during the 1960s and 1970s. She noted that, in these studies, the women represented the body in intrinsically physiological terms, particularly with reference to bodily image (face and eyes), but also with reference to those bodily parts with more 'erotic' connotations (flesh, skin, lips). Men, however, represented the body in material or functional terms (cells, machine) and referred to organic changes and concerns (death, accidents, pain). Furthermore, she described the women's representations of the body as having a 'euphoric tone', while the men were concerned with bodily potential. Comparing work conducted in 1963 and 1975, she noted a shift away from negative connotations to more pleasurable connotations of the body.

Research on body-image steadily increased from the 1980s. Grogan (2008) noted that this initially focused on women and girls, but increasingly it included men and boys. The focus on women reflected the greater concern with beauty, which has historically been linked with femininity. Bodily alterations designed to enhance beauty are widespread, even when these can pose a threat to health. One example of this is the use of tanning salons, which have grown in popularity since 2000. The 2010s was a time of recovery from the earlier economic depression, and consumer spending was on the rise in Britain. On the cultural scene, dance-pop music and artists like Lady Gaga grew in popularity. The first verse of her 2011 song *Born like this* starts, 'I'm beautiful in my way, "cause God makes no mistakes"' glorifying the importance of beauty in life.

In the early 2010s, a study of social representations of sun-bed tanning was conducted in England by Taylor et al. (2017). In this study, a sample of male and female tanners and non-tanners was interviewed about their use of tanning salons. Thematic analysis of the interview transcripts identified two primary dimensions: health and beauty. While both groups referred to the risky nature of tanning, the tanners attempted to protect themselves from the accusation of being vain and risk-taking by keeping their sun-tanning secret or asserting that they only used it sparingly. Some of the sun-tanners even went to the lengths of keeping the practice secret from family and friends, lest they think less of them. One woman who worked in a sun-tanning salon said: 'I mean to be honest I don't tend to tell people what my job is because I think that people will automatically not think very highly of me, erm, for it' (p. 164).

Many of the tanners underplayed the aesthetic aspects of sun-tanning, instead emphasizing its supposed health benefits. For example, some mentioned that they used the salon to obtain a 'base' before they went on holiday, thus protecting their skin from subsequent intense exposure. Others highlighted its value in alleviating skin conditions such as eczema.

Indeed, some even said that tanning was a secondary benefit of using a sun-bed, with the main objective being its health advantages. As one woman said: 'So the tanning side is not the main benefit, but it's a nice little "Brucie" bonus' (p. 166).

These defensive strategies used by the tanners highlighted the moral character of health in Western culture (Crawford, 2006). There is a certain tension between health and beauty in social representations. While the promotion of beauty is accepted, excessive promotion is seen as a reflection of a morally dubious person. For this reason, the sunbed users emphasized their limited use of sun-beds. Admittedly, while health is a positive attribute, excessive concern with health can also be a dubious practice, as seen in the development of hypochondriasis.

A second study examined the on-line posts regarding the use of sunbeds (Taylor et al., 2018). Once again, there was tension between health and beauty in the social representations of tanning. In the on-line discussion forums, the sun-bed non-users emphasized its health risks and characterized users as vain and preoccupied with their appearance. The sun-bed users defended their use on the grounds that they minimized any risks by limiting use, e.g., 'Yes, there are links to skin cancer, but I figure a couple of times a year can't hurt" (p. 529). They also mentioned its benefits in reducing subsequent exposure to intense sunlight, e.g., 'I used to burn when I was out in the sun now I don't burn at all because my skin has gotten used to tanning' (p. 530). This study illustrated the discursive and rhetorical strategies used by sun-bed users to protect themselves from the dominant negative social representation of sun-tanning as threatening to health.

5.6 Adults in 1990s Germany and Portugal

The 1990s was a period of dramatic change in Germany following the reunification of the country. After the Second World War, West Germany, operating under a capitalist model, had experienced sustained economic development with the establishment of a comprehensive health and social welfare system. East Germany had a Communist government for almost 50 years, and during this period, it also achieved substantial economic and social development despite sustained political repression (Hoyer, 2023). However, due to the accumulation of economic and political challenges, the East German government fell in 1989, and reunification followed.

It was within this context that a series of studies on social representations of health and illness were conducted by Uwe Flick.

Flick had trained in both psychology and sociology in Germany in the 1980s and then spent some time working with Moscovici in Paris in the early 1990s. He developed an interest in 'subjective theories' during his graduate work in Germany. These phenomenological theories are concerned with ways of thinking about the self and our everyday world. While in France, Flick contrasted these more person-centred German subjective theories with the more social French theories of social representations and edited a collection of empirical work from both traditions (Flick, 1993a).

In his introduction to the collection, Flick (1993b) referred to the influential work of Alfred Schutz (1899–1959), an Austrian philosopher who integrated ideas from phenomenology with those of such American psychologists as George Herbert Mead (1863–1931) and William James (1842–1910). In particular, Schutz was interested in the idea of intersubjectivity and how people grasp an understanding of each other in everyday life. This work provided Flick with a bridge to Moscovici's approach.

It was the social aspect of social representation theory that attracted Flick. The argument developed by Moscovici is that they develop in everyday social interaction but draw upon and contribute to broader social representations. As Flick stated:

> In the study of social representations, we favour, contrary to subjective theories, the individual-society relationship which is concretized in the relationship between subjective perception and the collective funds of knowledge on a theme (Flick, 1993b, p. 28, trans.).[2]

In addition, Flick was interested in the nature of qualitative research. In particular, he developed the concept of ***triangulation*** and the method of the ***episodic-interview***. Triangulation was an engineering concept derived from surveying and was concerned with using more than one approach to determine the character and location of something. This concept had been adopted by some social researchers to champion the use of different methods in the study of a particular phenomenon (Denzin, 1970). It was a strategy of validation. However, Flick emphasized that triangulation

[2] Dans l'étude des représentations sociales, on privilégie, à l'encontre des théories subjectives, la relation individu-société qui se concrétise dans la relation entre la perception subjective et les fonds collectifs de savoir sur un theme.

could consider not just different methods but also different theories and epistemologies (Flick, 1992). This 'strong' approach to triangulation was not just a simple combination of different methods but involved taking into consideration the strengths and weaknesses of the different theoretical perspectives.

As regards methods in qualitative research, Flick promoted the use of the episodic-interview. He felt that the standard interview encouraged the participant to talk in rather abstract terms about the phenomenon being investigated. He preferred using an episodic interview, which encouraged the participants to describe their everyday encounters with the phenomenon. In the same way, Mishler (1991) had criticized the standard interview researcher for ignoring the narrative content of interviews.

Flick (2000b) reported a series of studies he and his colleagues conducted on social representations of health and illness among different samples in Germany and Portugal. These studies used a similar method, involving interviews about what health meant to the study participants, followed by a request to provide a narrative account 'of situations in which the topic became relevant in the interviewee's actual everyday life of had become relevant in his or her biography' (p. 317). The interview transcripts were then subjected to intensive coding, which went through a series of stages from micro-themes to more macro-themes.

5.6.1 Nurses and Clerks in Germany

The first study comparing the social representations of health among East and West German nurses and clerks was conducted in 1994, shortly after reunification. The comparison of individuals from East and West Germany was designed to identify the role of the political context, while comparing nurses with clerks aimed to highlight the importance of a professional link to health. They developed a three-fold classification similar to that created by Herzlich (i.e., health in a vacuum, reserve of health and equilibrium) to describe the participants' representations of health, but augmented it with a category of health as lifestyle. This fourth category reflected a broader awareness of topics like nutrition, exercise and fitness.

Awareness of health was a central concept for organizing health conceptions. In the West, with a more differentiated health system, there was more 'reflexive dealing', while in the East, where there was greater centralized control, there was more suppression. In the West, there was more evidence of self-management (nurses) and alertness (clerks), while in the

East, there was more evidence of the need for control (nurses) and awareness of health (clerks).

There were also differences between the four groups of workers:

- Nurses from East Germany: need for control. This referred to the extent to which the person or the state had control over their health.
- Clerks from East Germany: awareness of health. This refers to health-related activities.
- Clerks from West Germany: scepticism leads to alertness. This ranged from scepticism about orthodox medicine to alertness regarding alternative ways of preventing illness.
- Nurses from West Germany: self-management of health. Health was seen as a result of one's own activities versus medical support.

Flick positioned the participants on the awareness dimension, starting with those highest in reflexive dealing—first the West German nurses, followed by the East German nurses, and then the West German clerks, followed by the East German clerks.

It was argued that these differences reflected the different healthcare systems in West and East Germany. In West Germany, the health system was very differentiated, requiring individuals to play an important role in seeking the type of healthcare, whereas the East German system was centralized, and individuals had less say in choosing the type of care. Also, in the West, there was greater emphasis on lifestyle, reflecting a more reflexive approach. They also noted the greater focus on awareness of health among the nurses, reflecting the importance of their deeper engagement with health issues and training.

Flick concluded that there is a double impact on the representations of health in the four groups due to the differences in the health systems experienced in 'the biographies and from the professional proximity to or distance from the topic of health' (p. 319). Thus, while the German participants had a similar social representation of health as the French participants in Herzlich's study, there were certain differences that reflected the character of German society and healthcare. The focus on lifestyle was a reflection of the growing influence of the health promotion focus of healthcare. It would seem that this was more dominant in West Germany, with its free enterprise consumerist culture. In East Germany, the greater role of the state overall placed more importance on the state as a provider of health.

5.6.2 *Women in Germany and Portugal*

The second study conducted by Flick and his colleagues contrasted the social representations of German and Portuguese women. These two countries not only have different languages but also different histories and healthcare regimes. Germany is a highly industrialized country with a developed health service, while Portugal is less industrialized with a developing health service. In addition, the two countries have different political histories.

A sample of women aged 28–36 years, half of whom had two or more children and had similar education levels, such as teachers, clerks or physiotherapists, participated in the study. These women were interviewed individually about their views on health and healthcare. The interview transcripts were subsequently coded.

The central difference between the two groups of women was the emphasis placed on the concept of awareness. In the interviews with the Portuguese women, the central theme was that of a lack of awareness, meaning it was felt that people did not take care of themselves, resulting in illness. It was felt that Portuguese people, in general, 'simply let things run' (p. 320). As one woman said: 'In my head, everything is there. But doing—it could be today, it could be tomorrow. It is today, tomorrow, and I will never do it' (p. 320). This lack of awareness was blamed on the state, which, it was felt, not only had poor infrastructure but also did not motivate people to care for their health.

This lack of awareness reflected a more general fatalism and resignation, which resulted from the long history of fascist governments in Portugal that were not overthrown until the Carnation Revolution of 1974. Conversely, among the German women, the central theme in their interviews was being 'forced to health'. This was due to residents feeling they had to be healthy and that those who became ill were treated as outsiders. As one woman said:

> ... the citizen is made an outsider by the media and the press and so on, is really forced to be in good shape. And the whole idea of health – who does not correspond to it, is an outsider then, as you are not accepted in our society in this way. A healthy, active, sportive human being is desired and is well accepted in the society. And people with an illness, they are marginalized, like AIDS, which is just an example (p. 321).

The women found this pressure to be healthily stressful. The pressure surrounded their everyday lives. As one woman said:

> Yes I think this obligation to health is indoctrinated to us, because we receive it from the media, we receive it from our surroundings, one almost could see it as global, we are permanently confronted with it. Who is fat is not good; who is ill is not good; who does not function is not good, disturbs the society in the end. I think the duty of a good citizen, that's what is trained to us and somehow becomes clear everywhere (p. 321).

The Portuguese women talked about a lack of awareness—*falta de cuidado*—meaning 'not to take care of oneself, not to be cautious for oneself'. They felt that this was the main cause of illness. This was linked to the public health system, which was seen as inadequate. The state was responsible because its lack of support for the health system was reflected in not motivating people to care for their health. It was suggested that a possible explanation was the history of military dictatorship in Portugal, resulting in a sense of fatalism and acceptance of fate.

The main focus of this study was on identifying the role of social, cultural and political factors in the development of different social representations of health. Flick concluded that the social representations of health were 'influenced by the concrete cultural, historical and social contexts in which they were made explicit' (p. 323). He added that the 'more general experiences with the health systems and changes in it are "anchored" in the health conceptions and "objectified" in specific metaphors—of awareness and control' (p. 323).

5.7 Health, Culture and Identity

Representations of health and illness develop out of everyday social interaction in particular cultural and historical contexts. Herzlich (1973) concluded her study with the remark, 'Health and illness thus appear as a mode of interpretation of society by the individual, and as a mode of relation of the individual to society' (p. 139). This is apparent in the different social representations of health and illness that were revealed in the various studies.

From a developmental perspective, adulthood is the period when young people begin to adopt certain adult roles and fulfil certain adult responsibilities within specific socio-cultural contexts. In Herzlich's study, health was seen as social action and engagement, and the participants strove to maintain this status. They felt ill if they were unable to do so.

In Blaxter's study, the working-class Scottish women stressed their moral worth by engaging in health protection activities. Similarly, in the study of working-class women in Northern Ireland, a central part of health was the health of the family and maintaining that health. The women positioned good motherhood as central to their identity. This positioning took place within a socio-cultural context in which motherhood was valued. In Stainton-Rogers' study, representations of health reflected the broader socio-political outlook. In Jovchelovitch and Gervais's study, Chinese participants portrayed their identity through their food practices. Finally, in Flick's studies, health action was conditioned by the broader political heritage of society.

In Herzlich's study, one of the dimensions of social representations of illness was conceptualized as liberation. This reflected the composition of her sample, which included people with health problems. In embodiment terms, the people with illness had experienced its benefits as freeing them from certain responsibilities, and this had become integrated into their social representation. In the other studies, there was little evidence of this dimension. Instead, the primary social representation of illness was as destruction. It destroyed your ability to engage in social activities, to work and to look after your family. People had a moral commitment to regain their health. This was the link with social identity as the study participants attempted to provide a certain coherence in their social representations. Their social representations of health in the various studies reflected the social identity of the participants in terms of gender, ethnicity and nationality but these are changing and the social representations accordingly.

From a historical perspective, these studies illustrate how the social representations of health and illness are tied to the changing social and political circumstances. While the 1960s was a period of recovery from the disruption and turmoil of the Second World War, Riley (2024) has identified the 1970s as the period when the search for health and well-being became more pronounced in Western society. It was also the period when there was sustained political upheaval and technological change. This search for health reflected a desire for a return to less frenetic times.

The centrality of equilibrium in social representations of health harks back to ancient ideas. In ancient Greece, *Harmonia* was the goddess of harmony and concord, who maintained a balance between conflict and peace. In Rome, her counterpart was *Concordia*. The term 'harmony' in music is concerned with the unity of different sounds. The ancient humoral model of health and illness considers health to be due to a balance of bodily humours while illness is due to an imbalance. It would seem that people were anchoring their representation of health and illness in these ancient ideas. The restoration of health required the restoration of this balance or equilibrium through diet and exercise. The pace of life in modern society was seen as a threat to this equilibrium. People could look back to their youth or to previous generations, when the pace of life was considered slower and, as a consequence, people were healthier. Rest and relaxation were key to slowing down the pace of life in the modern world, reflected in the frequent demand for more vacation time.

The social representations of health were anchored in those halcyon images of peace and tranquility. In the previous chapter, we mentioned the role of nostalgia as an explanation for the adoption of smoking by young people. Nostalgia for times past has been detailed by Arnold-Forster (2024) as a relatively modern phenomenon. It was first reported in the nineteenth century as a physical complaint experienced by people who were distant from their homes. However, in the modern era, it has become more of a psychological phenomenon, describing the experience of homesickness that could be for time as well as place. This nostalgia can be used by politicians and the media to conjure up a fantastic world that people have lost. This is a world where people are in balance with nature and where things move at a slower pace. This is *la vision rousseauiste* within which health is retrospectively anchored for many adults. Taylor (1991) in his critique of modernity contrasted this romantic perspective with the perspective of those who champion new technology. In this current time of change, people will not only connect social representations of health with past events but also with the future as represented in such artistic forms as literature, films and video games. The frequent use of biographical methods in the studies discussed provided participants with the opportunity to talk extensively about their lives and to locate the social representations in time and place. Future research will need to expand on these methods to further explore the changes in social representations.

References

Aim, M. -A., Decarsin, T., Bovina, I., & Dany, L. (2018). Health and social representations: A structural approach. *Papers on social representations, 27*(1), 1–21.

Arnold-Forster, A. (2024). *Nostalgia: A history of a dangerous emotion*. Picador.

Blatterer (2007). Contemporary adulthood: reconceptualizing an uncontested category. *Current Sociology*, 55(6), 771–792.

Blaxter, M. (1990). *Health and lifestyles*. Routledge.

Blaxter, M. (1993). Why do victims blame themselves? In A. Radley (Ed.), *Worlds of illness. Biographical and cultural perspectives on health and disease*. Routledge.

Blaxter, M., & Patterson, L. (1982). *Mothers and daughters: A three-generational study of health attributes and behaviour*. Heinemann.

Bousquet, G., & Pessin, A. (2003). Culture and identity in post-war France. In N. Hewitt (Ed.), *The Cambridge companion to modern French culture* (pp. 41–60). Cambridge University Press.

Canguilheim, G. (1943/1972). *Le normal et le pathologique (On the Normal and the Pathological)* [English translation] 1978, D. Reidel. Presses Universitaires de France.

Chabal, E. (2000). French political culture in the 1970s. Liberalism, identity politics and the modest state. *Geschichte Und Gesellschaft [History and Society]*, 42, 243–265.

Chrisafis, A. (2024, September 6). Macron defies the left by making Barnier PM. *The Guardian*, A1.

Crawford, R. (2006). Health as a meaningful social practice. *Health: An interdisciplinary journal for the social study of health, illness and medicine*, 10(4), 401–420.

Curt, B. C. (1994). *Textuality and tectonics. Troubling social and psychological science*. McGraw Hill.

d'Houtaud, A., & Field, M. G. (1984). The image of health: Variations in perception by social class in a French population. *Sociology of health and illness, 6*(1), 30–60.

Davies, P. (2001). *France and the second world war: Resistance, occupation and resistance*. Routledge.

Denzin, N. (1970). *The research act: A theoretical introduction to sociological methods*. McGraw-Hill.

Deschamps, J. C., & Guimelli, C. (2002). La composante émotionelle des représentations sociales: émotions rapportées et tendances à l'action dans une étude comparative des représentations sociales de l'insécurité en France et en Suisse. *Nouvelle Revue de Psychologie Sociale, 1*(1), 78–84.

Farr, R. M. (1977). Heider, Harré and Herzlich on health and illness: Some observations on the structure of 'representations collectives'. *European Journal of Social Psychology*, *7*(4), 491–504.
Finch, D., Wilson, H., & Bibby, J. (2023). Leave no one behind. In *The state of health and health inequalities in Scotland*. The Health Foundation.
Flick, U. (1992). Triangulation revisited: Strategy of validation or alternative? *Journal for the Theory of Social Behaviour*, 22(2), 175–192.
Flick, U. (ed.). (1993a). *La Perception Quotidienne de la Santé et de la Maladie. Théories Subjectives et Représentations Sociales*. L'Harmattan.
Flick, U. (1993b). La perception quotidienne de la santé et de la maladie. Aperçus général et introduction. In U. Flick (Ed.), *La Perception Quotidienne de la Santé et de la Maladie. Théories Subjectives et Représentations Sociales* (pp. 11–33). L'Harmattan.
Flick, U. (2000b). *Qualitative inquiries into social representations of health*.
Freidson, E. (1961–62). The sociology of medicine: A trend report and bibliography. *Current Sociology*, 3, 10–11.
Galland, O. (2008). Young people and society: Contrasting visions of the future. In A. Stellinger & R. Wintrebert (Eds.), *Young people facing the future—An international survey* (pp. 27–56). Foundation pour l'Innovation Politique.
Gergen, K.J., & Gergen, M.M. (1973). Narrative form and the construction of psychological science. In T. Sarbin(ed.), Narrative psychology: The storied nature of human conduct. Praeger.
Grogan, S. (2008). *Body image: Understanding body dissatisfaction among men, women and children* (2nd edn.). Taylor and Francis.
Guareschi, P. A., & Jovchelovitch, S. (2004). Participation, health and the development of community resources in Southern Brazil. *Journal of Health Psychology*, 9(2), 311–322.
Hale, R., Fox, C., & Murray, M. (2017). "As a parent you become a tiger": Parents talking about bullying at school. *Journal of Child and Family Studies*, *27*, 2000–2015.
Heaney, S. (1975). Whatever you say, say nothing. In S. Heaney (Ed.), *North* (pp. 57–60). Faber & Faber.
Heider, F. (1946). Attitudes and cognitive organization. *Journal of Psychology*, *21*(1), 107–112.
Heider, F. (1958). *The psychology of interpersonal relations*. John Wiley.
Herzlich, C. (1973). *Health and illness. A social psychological analysis*. Academic Press. (Original: *Santé et Maladie: Analyse d'une Réprésentation Sociale*. Paris: Mouton, 1969).
Herzlich, C., & Pierrer, J. (1984). *Illness and self in society*. Johns Hopkins University Press.
Herzlich, C. (1993). Réprésentations sociales de la santé et de la maladie et leur dynamique dans le champ social. In U. Flick (Ed.), *La Perception Quotidienne*

de la Santé et de la Maladie. Théories Subjectives et Représentations Sociales (pp. 11–33). L'Harmattan.

Herzlich, C. (2001). Les représentations sociales de la santé et la santé en mutation: Un regard rétrospectif et prospectif sur la fécondité d'un concept. In F. Buschini & N. Kalampalikis (Eds.), *Penser la vie, le Social, la nature. Mélanges en l'honneur de S. Moscovici* (pp. 189–200). Éditions de l'École des Hautes Études en Sciences Sociales.

Herzlich, C. (2018). A journey in the field of health: From social psychology to multi-disciplinarity. *Journal of Health Psychology, 23*, 386–396.

Hewitt, N. (2003). Introduction: French culture and society in the twentieth century. In N. Hewitt (Ed.), *The Cambridge companion to modern French culture* (pp. 1–16). Cambridge University Press.

Hoyer, K. (2023). *Beyond the wall. East Germany, 1949–1990*. Allen Lane.

Jodelet, D. (1984). Représentation sociale: Phénomènes, concept et théorie. In S. Moscovici (Ed.), *Psychologie Sociale* (pp. 357–378). Presses Universitaires de France.

Jovchelovitch, S., & Gervais, M. C. (1999). Social representations of health and illness: The case of the Chinese community in England. *Journal of Community and Applied Social Psychology, 9*, 247–260.

László, J. (1997). Narrative organization of social representations. Papers on Social Representations, 6.2, 154–167.

Mishler, E. G. (1991). *Research interviewing. Context and narrative*. Harvard University Press.

Moscovici, S. (1961). *La Psychanalyse: Son Image et Son Public*. Presses Universitaires de France.

Moscovici, S. (1998). Social consciousness and its history. *Culture and Psychology*, 4(3), 411–429.

Moscovici, S. ([1976] 2008). *Psychoanalysis: Its image and its public* [English translation of La psychoanalyse, son image et son image, 1976]. Polity Press.

Moscovici, S., & Marková, I. (1998). Presenting social representations: A conversation. *Culture and Psychology*, 4(3), 371–410.

Murray, M., & McMillan, C. (1988). *Working class women's views of health, illness and the health service*. Prepared for Ulster Cancer Foundation.

Murray, M. (2002). Connecting narrative and social representation theory in health research. *Social Science Information*, 41(4), 653–673.

Pill, R., & Stott, N. (1985). Choice or chance: Further evidence on ideas of illness and responsibility for health. *Social Science and Medicine*, 20(10), 881–191.

Pitti, I. (2017). What does being an adult mean? Comparing young people's and adults' representations of adulthood. *Journal of Youth Studies, 20*(9), 1225–1241.

Porch, D. (2024). *Resistance and liberation. France at war, 1942–1945*. Cambridge University Press.

Proust, M. (2022). *Sur le bon usage des mauvaises santés*. ORMA.

Riley, J. (2024). *Well beings: How the seventies lost its mind and taught us to find ourselves*. Icon Books.
Sartre, J. -P. ([1943] 2020). *Being and nothingness. An essay in phenomenological ontology*. Routledge.
Stainton-Rogers, W. (1991). *Explaining health and illness. An exploration of diversity*. Harvester Wheatsheaf.
Stenner, P., Watts, S., & Worrell, M. (2008). Q methodology. In C. Willig & W. Stainton-Rogers (Eds.), *The SAGE handbook of qualitative research in psychology* (pp. 215–239). Sage.
Stoetzel (1960). La maladie, le malade et le médecin: esquisse d'une analyse psychosociale.Population, 15 (4),613–624.
Sulivan, J. (2000). *Anticipate every goodbye* (E. Maher, Trans.). Veritas.
Taylor, C. (1991). The ethics of authenticity. Harvard University Press.Wallston, B.S., & Wallston, K.A. (1978). Locus of control: A review of the literature. Health Education Monographs, 6, 107–116.
Taylor, J., Lamont, A., & Murray, M. (2018). Talking about sunbed tanning in online discussion forums: Assertions and arguments. *Psychology and Health*, 33 (4), 518–536.
Taylor, J., Murray, M., & Lamont, A. (2017). Talking about sunbed use: Social representations, identity and resistance. *Social Science and Medicine*, 184, 161–168.
Townsend, P., & Davidson, N. (1982). *Inequalities in health: The black report*. Penguin.
Wallston, K. A., Wallston, B. S., & DeVellis, R. (1978). Development of the multidimensional health locus of control (MHLC) scales. *Health Education Monographs*, 6(2), 160–170.

CHAPTER 6

Infectious Diseases, Cancer and Mental Illness

While adulthood is characterized as a period of health and well-being, it is also a period when people begin to confront certain serious health problems, both among themselves, their family and the wider community. Most feared are those conditions that seem to be resistant to treatment, such as new infectious diseases and cancer, as well as mental illness. These three health problems are extensive. In the case of infectious diseases, two new conditions have recently emerged—HIV/AIDS and COVID-19. In the case of cancer, the condition impacts different parts of the body and has different effects on life expectancy. Finally, mental illness is a term that describes a wide range of cognitive and emotional challenges. This chapter considers the different social representations of these conditions and places them in their socio-historical context.

6.1 Infectious Diseases

All previous societies have experienced mass scourges of infectious diseases. They were mass phenomena that impacted whole societies, against which little could be done, leading inevitably to death for many and against which the only protection was through exclusion of the afflicted. Over time, these diseases steadily declined after causing widespread death and destruction.

M. Murray, *Social Representations, Health and Illness*,
https://doi.org/10.1007/978-3-031-98494-5_6

6.1.1 *Historic Images of Infectious Diseases*

Leprosy is an early example of an infectious disease. It was frequently mentioned in the Bible and other ancient texts (Alpert, 2024). For example, the apostle Mark wrote in his gospel about an encounter Jesus had with a person with leprosy: 'And a leper came to him, imploring him, and kneeling said to him, "If you will, you can make me clean." Moved with pity he stretched out his hand and touched him and said to him, "I will; be clean", And immediately the leprosy left him and he was made clean' (Mark, 1:40–41). This miraculous treatment of the disease reflects the historic linkage of moral transgressions with disease.

With the rise of infectious diseases in the Middle Ages, leprosy began to be more widely discussed in Western literature. Houston (2016) has traced the changing literary representations in England between the 1200s and 1600s. She noted how it changed from a disease that was considered a sign of holy suffering and nearness to God to a physical indication of a diseased and sinful soul. Leprosy is, at first, a hidden disease until it takes over and destroys the body. Historically, the management of the disease was limited to the isolation of the afflicted, who were excluded from communities and required to signal their presence with a cry or a rattle.

Although leprosy impacted individuals, the plague affected entire communities. The afflicted died in miserable conditions. The only hope to avoid the disease, once the plague arrived in a community, was to flee. Fear and panic were widespread reactions to the arrival of the plague. Often, the very word 'plague' was avoided, and various euphemisms were used instead. Additionally, the term was used to describe other threatening events. Rather than causing alarm, some individuals adopted a more fatalistic approach and reacted to the onset of the plague with a degree of equanimity. It was God's will. In Arnold Bocklin's (1827–1901) painting *Plague* (1898), the disease is portrayed as an evil marauder roaming the streets. The very popular image of death as the Grim Reaper, with his scythe seeking more unfortunate victims, is frequently depicted in religious paintings.

Albert Camus, in his classic existentialist novel *The Plague* (Camus, 1947), described the impact of a plague sweeping through a French Algerian town. He began by quoting from the earlier account *A Journal of the Plague Year* (1722) by the English writer Daniel Defoe: 'It is as reasonable to represent one kind of imprisonment by another, as it is to represent anything that really exists by that which exists not'—a kind of reverse objectification. Camus vividly described the growing fear as the plague spread throughout the city. Through certain characters, he detailed the different reactions, from those who took advantage of the plague to those who tried to help others. One of the characters, Joseph Grand, who was trying to write a novel, volunteered to help. Reflecting on this altruism, Camus wrote optimistically at the close that 'there is more to admire in humans than to scorn'. The saintly image of the person assisting those impacted by infectious diseases remains.

Eventually, the plague died out in the eighteenth century, to be replaced by cholera and then tuberculosis. The French writer Chateaubriand, writing about the 1832 cholera epidemic, compared it with the 1720 plague in Marseilles: 'Half-rotted corpses lay amidst mud-soaked rags; others stood leaning against the walls in the position in which they had expired' (Herzlich & Pierret, 1980, p. 7). Another feature noted in the 1832 cholera epidemic was the role of spectators, who watched with horror and fascination as the afflicted were carried away. Each epidemic had its time course; some ravaged the individual rapidly, while others slowly consigned the individual to inevitable death.

In the nineteenth century, the major fear was directed at tuberculosis, which accounted for as many as a quarter of all deaths in Europe during that century. This disease was first detected among the wealthy and was assumed to reflect a condition of both passion and refinement. An association with art and literature evolved, as those affected were assumed to have a creative imagination. Treatment was largely in terms of rest and confinement, initially at home and then in special sanatoria, which were often located in scenic mountainous locations. Altitude, fresh air, exercise and fatty food were the key components of treatment in these sanitoria (Kaptein et al., 2020). There remained a certain fear about contact with the afflicted.

This image of a disease of passion was reflected in literary representations, with several novels portraying rest in sanitoria as the best treatment. The most famous of these novels is *The Magic Mountain* (1924) by Thomas Mann (1875–1955), in which the central character visits a colleague in a Swiss sanatorium and develops tuberculosis. He remains there, and the novel is a reflection upon many issues, including illness and death. The contemporary image of the sanitorium as an uncertain place of refuge is conveyed in the novel *The Empusium* (2024) by the Polish novelist Olga Tokarczuk. The book, which is sub-titled *A Health Resort*

Horror Story, details the continuing fear of these institutions. The central character in the novel is sent to a sanatorium, where he dreads being watched, and the fear of death fills the book.

As the disease spread throughout Europe, it became more associated with poverty. It was not a disease of wealth but more of penury and deprivation. In paintings, the link between tuberculosis and poverty is commonplace. For example, in *The Sick Child* (1885) by Edvard Munch (1863–1944), the patient with tuberculosis is painted as emaciated and otherworldly—due to poverty and possibly excessive passion. Thus, there were these two conflicting images of the disease: one of refinement and the other of poverty.

By the end of the nineteenth century, any resignation in the face of death had become less apparent, especially among the more affluent, who were beginning to enjoy the benefits of longevity due to improved living conditions. Furthermore, with the development of medical science, illness began to be conceived more in biological terms. However, for the masses of the nineteenth century, sickness and death were still accepted as part of life.

Despite the improvements in living conditions and healthcare, new infectious diseases continue to emerge in different parts of the world. The development of social representations of these new diseases often draws on images from past epidemics, illustrating their historical character.

6.1.2 HIV/AIDS

HIV (human immunodeficiency virus) is a virus that attacks the immune system, leading to the development of AIDS (acquired immunodeficiency syndrome). Evidence for the existence of AIDS first became apparent in the early 1980s. After a sustained program of biomedical research, the virus, which is spread by sexual contact or through infected blood, was identified in 1983, and the search began for effective treatment.

In the 1980s, there was no effective treatment for AIDS, and the incidence rate continued to rise. In the early years, the disease was largely confined to three groups: gay and bisexual men, people who injected drugs, and people with haemophilia receiving blood products. By the 1990s, there was evidence of increasing incidence among women. The rate continued to increase until 2005, when treatment became more effective and the diagnosis was no longer a death sentence. Governments launched a mass media campaign to prevent the spread of the disease.

When it was first identified, this disease created sustained alarm in the Western world as there was no known cure, and it was usually followed by the early death of those afflicted. Since its initial detection until 2022, it has been estimated that HIV/AIDS has led to almost 40 million deaths globally (UNAIDS, 2022). These deaths were particularly concentrated in Eastern and Southern Africa. Subsequently, effective treatment through suppression of the virus has been developed. Although there is currently no total cure for HIV, it is still possible for HIV+ people to lead a relatively normal life by following a detailed drug regimen. A series of studies have charted the public reaction to this new infectious disease.

The arrival of this new infectious disease was met with alarm in the Western media. The focus was on the threat posed by this new disease. An early study of the portrayal of HIV/AIDS in the UK media (Marková and Wilkie, 1987) emphasized that the public reaction to the threat was not simply a cognitive reaction but also an emotional one. The disease was seen as a moral disease and as a punishment for sexual irresponsibility. In an early report in *The Times*, a reporter remarked: 'It does not need anyone's backing to see that most AIDS victims will be the results of their own irresponsibility' (*The Times*, 24.1.1987). This was similar to how venereal disease was represented in the nineteenth century. In both cases, the government reacted by championing a conservative sexual campaign as a means of curtailing the spread of the disease. Marková and Wilkie noted the anchoring of both AIDS and syphilis in death, 'improper' sexual behaviour and 'just' punishment. This was the dominant view in the early stages of the AIDS epidemic but was challenged by minority groups.

This context is important, as the origin of social representations is often derived from scientific representations of the phenomenon, which are conveyed to the public via the media and various official documents. However, this is not a one-way process; rather, some of the early scientific ideas themselves develop from still-evolving lay ideas and also from ancient and mythical ideas about the causes of various threats. The earliest accounts of AIDS reflected public anxiety, and it was labelled Gay-Related Immune Deficiency before the virus was identified and it was seen to have spread beyond the gay community.

Anchoring HIV/AIDS in South Africa: South Africa was a major 'hot spot' for HIV/AIDS compared with the UK. In 1990/91, when the rate of HIV/AIDS was continuing to increase, Joffe (1996b) conducted a study of the social representations of the disease. A total of 60 adults, drawn from the two countries, participated in the study. These participants were gay men and heterosexual men and women from Black and White communities. They were interviewed about the disease, and the interview transcripts were coded. In addition, Joffe conducted a systematic review of the government HIV/AIDS prevention campaigns to provide an understanding of the context within which the participants developed their social representations.

In terms of objectification, Joffe noted that the disease was represented in media campaigns using threatening images such as tombstones and coffins. The lay participants extended these images and talked about five main causes: aberrant sexuality (including bestiality and promiscuity), tribal rituals (including cannibalism and incest), 'Third World' factors (such as lack of Western medicine and overcrowded living conditions), unhygienic practices and the practices of uneducated people. A 'sin cocktail' was a combination of two or more of these causal factors. An example is the comment by a British White heterosexual male:

> Monkeys in Africa. I think that was what I heard and that was passed through God knows what to get through. I've heard some extreme stories about how it reached our shore [much laughter]. Which I dare not to utter... It was just meant to be bestiality, I suppose (Joffe, 1996b, p. 180).

Conversely, a South African Black heterosexual male said:

> As I heard it started in England... It started between a monkey and a person after a person intercoursing with a monkey... after the person intercoursing with the monkey he never washed and he went to his partner (Joffe, 1996b, p. 181).

These aberrant images were drawn upon to make this new phenomenon concrete.

In discussing the disease, the participants anchored the disease in the 'other'. The 'other' depended upon the group perceived as threatened. The White participants attributed the cause of HIV/AIDS to activities in Africa, whereas Black participants attributed it to activities in the West. Furthermore, a third of the participants felt that they were not threatened by the disease since they were not part of a certain out-group (e.g., homosexuals). As one British Black heterosexual male said:

> It is like word association, isn't it? I think about AIDS I think of drug use, I think of decadent Stars, I think of homosexuals. I very rarely think of heterosexuals when I think about it (Joffe, 1996b, p. 179).

This attribution to the 'other' was similar to the dominant images of the disease in the mass media at that time.

In anchoring the disease to the 'other', the group is protected from the threat. However, for some people, this negative causal attribution may be to the self or the in-group. This is a version of Goffman's (1963) 'spoiled identity' thesis. The adoption of which of these orientations—to the out-group or to the in-group—depends upon the dominance differential between the in-group and the other. Where the in-group is devalued, the causal attribution can be to the in-group's negative behaviours. Many gay men had internalized a negative view of their own group. As one British Black gay man said:

> I am gay myself, but gay people are so damned disgusting. Um, you've got, I mean, let's not beat about the bush here ... the element is so strong whereby by now we are living in an age where a man will approach a man in broad daylight ... there's a lot of deviant behaviour going on (Joffe, 1996b, p. 182).

Rather than internalize the cause of the disease, gay groups increasingly adopted a more resistant stance. The spoiled identity could be challenged through forms of identity management, which could inject minority ideas into existing representations. The ability of the minority group to exercise such influence depended upon their power relationship. While the gay voice in Britain was unified and influential in the media, in South Africa, it was more fragmented and less powerful. In Britain, a cohesive minority group was able to challenge the dominant social representation and assert a view of safe sex rather than one of conservative moral values.

Joffe (1996a, 1999) extended the discussion of othering by considering potential psychodynamic processes. According to the child psychoanalyst Klein (1946), the psychodynamic process of 'splitting' develops at an early age in children. It is a process of protecting the self from external threats by splitting the world into either good or bad. The aim of splitting is to protect the good self from the bad. Joffe extended this approach from the individual to the group. Thus, when the group encounters a threat, it exacerbates the splitting defence and the consequent out-group blaming mechanism. The extent to which this mechanism can operate depends upon the social heritage of the group and the current social order.

Overall, the study illustrated the processes by which social representations grasp a new disease, how it is objectified and anchored in the 'other'. It also illustrated the nature of conflicting explanations as being both due to immoral behaviour and to not taking precautions. Furthermore, consideration of the social identity of the impacted group illustrated the role of the cohesive minority in challenging dominant social representations.

Telling stories about HIV/AIDS in Africa: In a series of studies in Africa, Kate Winskell and colleagues (e.g., Beres et al., 2013; Winskell, 2021) explored young people's creative narratives about HIV/AIDS. Between 1997 and 2014, 150,000 young people across sub-Saharan Africa participated in a script writing exercise about HIV. They were asked to develop a creative idea about HIV that could be used for a short film. This created an archive of approximately 75,000 narratives about the disease (www.globaldialogues.org). Winskell et al. (2020) have conducted an analysis of over 1000 of these narratives, looking at both their context and how they are structured. In examining these narrative accounts, Winskell emphasized that they were fictional accounts and thus provided particular access to the young people's social representations of the disease.

The aim of the project was to encourage young people to reflect upon this threat through the development of a fictional film script (Winskell & Enger, 2014). Winskell (2021) later reflected that 'although fictional stories are invented depictions of social fact, they are still culturally-determined social facts in and of themselves and are, as Rabinow (1986) describes, a source of insight into how people make sense of the worlds, and how they communicate those understandings to others in their cultural community' (p. 169). They are also part of a collective action designed to transform their world. The subsequent use of the videos provides an opportunity for discussion and debate about how to control the HIV epidemic.

With such a massive corpus of narrative accounts, they were able to distinguish between the social representations of HIV that were dominant in different socio-cultural contexts. For example, they found that the othering of the source of the infection and a preoccupation with its circumstances were more common in lower-prevalence countries. They found that the most moralizing narratives were more apparent in those countries in which evangelical Protestant movements were strong.

In Swaziland, which has a high prevalence of HIV, the tone of the narratives was less one of tragedy and more one of resilience and agency, suggesting that the country has developed cultural resources to cope with the disease. The use of condoms mentioned in these narrative accounts revealed the more hegemonic representations of gender. Condom negotiation was more frequently initiated by women but rejected by men as threatening their masculinity.

In a detailed analysis of a small sample of these narratives, they found certain conflicts and contradictions in their accounts. They suggested that this was evidence of the operation of cognitive polyphasia and the co-existence of traditional and more scientific models of the disease. Winskell et al. (2013) noted the connection between the narrative accounts and the social representations of HIV. These narrative accounts were produced by individuals, but they drew upon the broader social representations and were also constrained by cultural narrative prototypes in terms of tone and structure. Furthermore, it can be argued that the young people were actively involved in the process of objectification through the narrative construction of accounts about HIV. The disease was not some abstract phenomenon but was enmeshed in cultural and personal resources through which narrative accounts were constructed.

6.1.3 COVID-19

COVID-19 is a major infectious disease caused by the coronavirus SARS-CoV-2. The disease leads to fever, respiratory problems and, in severe cases, to death. It was first identified in China in 2019 and then spread rapidly around the globe. National governments introduced a variety of measures to curtail the spread of this pandemic. The restrictions included the wearing of masks in public and limiting social interaction. This led to major social and economic disruption. In 2020, several vaccines were developed, which were quickly introduced. Eventually, the pandemic was brought under control, but not before over seven million deaths were recorded worldwide (WHO, 2025).

COVID-19 in the media: According to the polling agency IPSOS, COVID-19 emerged as the most feared disease in a survey of 31 countries in 2020 and remained so for two years (IPSOS, 2024). Newspapers throughout the world carried details of the spread of the disease. A study of three mainstream newspapers in the United States, Britain and China was conducted by Ittefaq et al. (2022). They identified four main themes: *the racialization of the virus* as a multi-faceted threat, COVID-19 *disease as a threat*, calls for *collective action* to curb the racialization of the virus and *speculative solutions* to end discrimination against Asians. The *racialization of the virus* occurred in a period of growing nationalism and global recession, 'triggering xenophobic reactions and behaviors such as discrimination, hate crimes, and harassment against Chinese individuals' (p. 19). It also occurred in the 'tension-fraught political sphere' of conflict between the West and China.

The *disease as a threat* theme grew in importance due to the difficulty governments faced in controlling the spread of the virus. It was suggested that it might have contributed to people seeking out other sources of information and the growth of conspiracy theories. It may also have contributed to people being reluctant to socialize, except with like-minded individuals, as a form of protection.

The third and fourth themes were a *call for collective action* to curb the racialization of the virus and to end discrimination against Asians. This was an indication of some media's urge to promote a sense of community to combat the disease and challenge racial tension. Newspapers adopted an action-oriented approach both socially and politically. However, it was noted that specific solutions for combatting racism were rarely identified. These media representations of COVID-19 contributed to an emotional response from readers, leading to anxiety and negative actions against Chinese people, who were identified as the cause of the disease.

The media plays an important role in the construction of social representations of the disease. Locating the cause of the disease in China was a means of 'thematic anchoring'. It not only provided a simple explanation for the disease but could potentially lead to action against the threat. The frequent references in the media to Chinese dietary habits and wet markets provided visual anchors, which reinforced the outsider message. This negative image was combined with the scientific message conveyed by government experts, leading to cognitive polyphasia, where people could hold conflicting messages. The emotional content of the racialized message also drew upon broader images of the unhygienic foreigner.

Conflicting images of COVID-19 are evident in the many photographs presented in news reports. A BBC report presented a collection of these images (BBC, 2020). This included images of empty streets, people clapping for the NHS and rainbow paintings of support for health workers, combined with photographs of patients in intensive care and people receiving the vaccine. Together, they portrayed the threat posed by the virus, leading to social isolation and mask-wearing as the primary means of protection. This was coupled with images of action by the government to combat the disease through both treatment and vaccination. These images contributed to the social representation of the disease as threatening but which we all could be involved in combatting. It coupled the prevention of the disease with the image of the good citizen, similar to that of the good mother mentioned in Chap. 6.

Learning to fear COVID in Spain: The disease not only affected adults but also children. One study conducted in the Basque area of Spain in the 2010s was interesting both methodologically and practically (Idoiaga et al., 2020). In this study, the parents of 250 children aged 3–12 years were approached to collect information from the children in a free-association exercise. The parents acted as interviewers and asked their children two questions: (1) 'These days we are talking a lot about the coronavirus. When you hear the word coronavirus, what comes to mind, what do you think?' and (2) 'How are you feeling these days because of the coronavirus?' The parents were asked to write down precisely what their child said without changing the words in any way.

The children's responses to the two questions were then subjected to lexical analysis. This produced two primary themes or clusters, which were labelled *coronavirus* and *lockdown*. The coronavirus theme consisted of two classes—*Our enemy, the virus* and *fear of contagion*. A typical comment categorized in the enemy class was:

> It's a virus but we don't really know what it is. We have to stay home and beat it because it's bad and it's a bug or something that gets into our tummy. In the street the doctors, who are heroes and brave, are going to beat it and that's why we go out every afternoon to the balcony to clap for them.

A typical comment in the class concerning fear of contagion was:

> It's a virus but since it's new we're all a little scared and they talk about it on the radio, on television and everywhere else. It doesn't hurt children but we can infect our grandparents and that scares me and that's why we can't go to their house.

The lockdown theme contained two linked classes—*safe at home* and *emotions regarding lockdown*—and a third class—*When is this going to end?* A typical comment from the 'safe at home' class was: 'The virus can't get into my house so I am happy here and I don't want to go out. Besides, I am happy to play with my family a lot'. The 'emotions' theme contained a mix of positive (happy and cheerful with family) and negative comments (bored, angry, overwhelmed, tired and lonely). The final class concerned frustration about the length of the pandemic and included comments like: 'I have doubts because I don't know when this boring confinement is going to end. I want to go back to school and play with my friends'.

A lexical analysis of the emotion-related words revealed the centrality of fear, which was mainly concerned with them infecting their grandparents. The children were frightened of leaving the safety of their homes, where they felt happy, although sometimes bored. The threat was something outside their homes. They could be good children by staying at home.

COVID 'othering' in Brazil: Social representations not only provide a framework for managing threats, but they also contribute to the development of dominant discourses in society. This was apparent in a study in Brazil conducted during the early stages of the COVID-19 pandemic (Souza et al., 2021). Brazil is a society with massive social inequalities, which are reflected not only in living conditions and health status but also in the provision of healthcare. It was one of the countries most highly affected by the disease. A small sample of 13 middle-class Brazilians was interviewed in depth about the disease. The interview transcripts were thematically analysed. Three primary categories were inductively identified, each of which had a number of sub-categories.

The first category considered COVID an *anthropocentric virus* whose transmission centred on human action. It included concern about: (a) the destruction of the environment and virus mutations, (b) the practices and intentions of the Chinese and (c) the spiritual or divine origin of the virus. The focus here was on the negative human actions that contributed to the development of the virus. The second category viewed COVID as a *dramatic virus.* This included: (a) the uncontrollable spread of the virus and the fragile victims and (b) the attack on the lungs and the undignified death. The focus of this category was on the immediate serious consequences of the virus, leading to a 'terrible and desperate disease'.

The third category was COVID as a *crisis* serving to improve mankind. This included: (a) a tragedy that threatens global health and alters daily life, (b) a correction and learning event and (c) the causes and meanings of the pandemic. This category focused more on the implications for mankind. On the one hand, it threatened life on this planet, but it also was a possible divine intervention to correct immoral behaviours and offered an opportunity for human beings to reassess their life trajectory.

The primary ideological implication of this social representation was the focus on the individual, and in particular, their moral correctness, mental strength and maturity. This, in turn, would aid in the blaming of socially disadvantaged groups who were perceived as lacking in moral correctness. The pandemic was part of a moral reform of mankind, focusing on the failings of the disadvantaged. The good people would be saved. There was also an alignment with dominant anti-Chinese attitudes in the identification of China as the source of the virus due to their aberrant eating practices. The objectification of the virus was evident in the images used to refer to its origin (the destruction of the forests, crowded cities full of waste, the food in China), the nature of the virus (an anthropocentric entity) and the nature of the disease (drowning in water, burials with plastic bags).

The dramatic representation of the disease also promoted an 'othering' of it, such that these middle-class participants could feel protected from it. They were morally upright and kept their environment clean. Those who were vulnerable were the disadvantaged and the irresponsible youth, who were feckless. The pandemic would serve to improve society. This study demonstrated the bottom-up process in the construction of ideology. The victim-blaming images in the social representations of these middle-class participants affirmed the dominant conservative ideological discourse and enabled political leaders to evade concern about structural inequalities as important causal agents.

In their analysis, Souza et al. (2021) adopted what they described as a phenomenological approach. This was designed to consider each participant individually as well as collectively. This was similar to the clinical case approach adopted by Herzlich (1973), such that they were able to see how the various descriptions of the disease were connected.

6.2 Cancer

Cancer is a term used to describe a group of diseases in which cell growth is uncontrolled and can spread to different parts of the body, leading to a variety of symptoms and possibly death. The IPSOS (2024) survey confirmed that cancer was the most feared disease in Britain in 2018 and remained so until it was replaced for two years (2020–22) by COVID-19. This fear was especially high among baby-boomers and women. Sontag (1977) suggested that this fear of the disease reflected a broader fear of death, especially a slow death, in modern society. She noted that the very term cancer has entered into everyday discourse as a metaphor for evil.

6.2.1 Artistic Images of Cancer

Historic images: Although cancer is often considered a modern disease, there is evidence from various sources that it has been present in various forms for thousands of years. Written records of the disease have been discovered in several ancient civilizations, such as Egypt and Greece (Hajdu, 2010). Also, since at least medieval times, there have been portrayals of cancer in art. Breast cancer is the form of cancer that has been represented in several paintings. Vaidya (2007) has described portrayals of breast cancer in paintings by Raphael and Leonardo da Vinci and noted that the women in these early paintings were often young, a feature of contemporary social representations of the disease.

In the nineteenth century, the widespread fear of tuberculosis was replaced by the fear of cancer. It was not the most common cause of death, which was heart disease, but its hidden character made it more feared. Patterson (1987) noted that a silence about cancer was present in nineteenth-century America, reflecting widespread anxiety. He identified three aspects of this fear of cancer:

1. It characterized life itself in the sense that, as a runaway growth, it mimicked normal development as if some cruel mockery of human pretensions.
2. It was perceived as an alien invader that gave little or no warning before eating into people.
3. It had a sinister aspect, tearing into the flesh and 'often ravaging one's private organs and leaving victims feeling dirty, betrayed by their bodies, without control over themselves'.

Patterson (1987) also suggested that today, in our more secular age, with the substantial improvements in people's living standards, the threat posed by cancer and death has become more magnified. No longer is death accepted or even welcomed; instead, it is fought. The major agent in this 'war against cancer' has been medicine.

The nineteenth century saw the development of modern anxiety about the disease in Britain, becoming 'a potent metaphor for anything evil, malevolent, or menacing' (Arnold-Foster, 2021, p. 55). It was during the Victorian period, with the rise of medicine, that cancer was portrayed as a major threat. This led to the growth of dedicated hospitals for patients with cancer and the search for a biomedical cure.

Cancer in the media: Cancer is a frequent topic of interest in the media. In a study of health-related articles published in Canadian magazines in 1991, 1996, and 2001, it was found that breast cancer was the most frequently discussed cancer (Clarke & Everest, 2006). A manifest analysis, which considered the explicit content of the articles, revealed that the medical framing was most common, followed by lifestyle and political economy. They identified three latent or hidden themes: (i) the exacerbation of fear, (ii) contradictions and uncertainty about diagnosis and treatment and (iii) frequent use of battle metaphors. Fear was the most dominant theme, and it was heightened in various ways: (i) conflation of cancer with fear, (ii) description of the disease growing silently, (iii) emphasis on increasing rates of the disease, (iv) portrayal of cancer as almost inevitable, (v) association of cancer with normal experience, (vi) association of fear with cancer screening and (vii) use of scary statistics.

Biomedicine was the dominant frame for explaining cancer, but it was also a source of fear. Medical doctors were frequently quoted, and there was limited reference to other professionals, such as epidemiologists or public health practitioners. Thus, there was limited reference to political economy as a source of the disease. It was concluded that 'the medical framing of the disease reflects the most powerful and wealthiest interests such as those of highly successful industries such as manufacturing pharmaceuticals and medical devices' (p. 2598). This medical framing of the disease is reflected in the focus on screening as the primary approach for the early detection of the disease (Kearney & Murray, 2009).

Cancer stories: Cancer is a frequent focus of attention in art and literature. In the classic nineteenth-century novel *The Death of Ivan Ilyich* (1886) by Lev Tolstoy (1828–1910), the central character, a former judge, develops cancer. He describes the suffering he endures, which he terms 'inexpressible'. In Thomas Mann's more modern account, *The Black Swan* (1953), a middle-aged woman develops cancer. Mann vividly describes the impact: 'the extinction of her physical womanhood, to whose spasmodic progress she responded with repeated psychological resistance. It induced states of anxiety, emotional unrest, headaches, days of depression, and an irritability' (in von Engelhardt, 2021).

The phenomenological descriptions in literature of the suffering experienced by the cancer patient were combined with reflections on the reactions of other people to the diagnosis. In his review of the wide-ranging literary representations of cancer, von Engelhardt (2021) described it as veering between the experience of the patient and the social reaction to the disease. It conveyed the image of a hidden evil, which heightened the fear of the disease.

One of the most popular contemporary literary genres is that of people who have experienced and overcome some traumatic event. In Western society, autobiographical accounts have been written about such events as sexual assault, depression and other psychological conditions, as well as more specific diseases such as heart disease and cancer. The extensive nature of this literature has given rise to the term 'pathography' as a descriptor of the genre (Hawkins, 1993). A review of a collection of novels and autobiographies about different types of cancer identified four main themes: *giving meaning to cancer, coping with medical treatment and the psychological* and *social consequences of the disease* (Kaptein, 2021).

One particular subset of this genre is the large number of books written by women about the experience of breast cancer. An exploration of the content of a selection of these accounts published in the 1990s (Murray, 2009) confirmed that this disease was especially feared by women because of its seemingly random nature and the fact that it seemed to strike women in the prime of their lives. This fear would seem to be heightened by the fact that it impacted the breast, the physical centre of femininity. As Comfort (1992) wrote about getting breast reconstruction after surgery: 'At age thirty-eight, I felt I was too young to be flat-chested for the rest of my life. I wanted my body to have some feminine curves' (p. 12).

A key aspect of the threat posed by breast cancer was its potential danger to a woman's life. The women emphasized that they were prepared to challenge this threat to their lives. The metaphor of a battle has an extremely wide currency with respect to the treatment of cancer (Sontag, 1977). In the women's accounts, the battle was usually in collaboration with medicine or various alternative remedies. For some women, this battle took on religious overtones.

The second theme in the breast cancer accounts was that of unpreparedness and undeservedness. This reflected a belief in the random character of cancer. Heart disease is considered to be caused by lifestyle, and so the victim bears some responsibility, in the case of breast cancer, it seemed to strike young, healthy, blameless people. Pinell (1987), in her analysis of letters written by cancer patients, made a similar comment about the blameless stance adopted by the authors. She argued that this stance of innocence is a requirement for subsequently expressing a critical discourse with regard to dominant negative representations.

One popular strategy to combat the disease was to focus on the positive. Many of the women were self-consciously aware of this strategy. For example, Wadler (1992) felt that she had to try to adopt a positive outlook but found that this strategy held within it many problems. She recalled: 'If there is a chance positive thinking can work, I feel I should try it, but I'm sceptical. If being a worrier has contributed to this disease, am I going to be able to alter my personality quickly enough to stop it?'

The women were aware of the negative image of cancer and wanted to avoid being discredited by others. The two strategies of impression management suggested by Goffman (1963) were apparent in the women's accounts. He distinguished between discredited and discreditable identities. In the discreditable situation, the individual concerned has the opportunity to pass as normal, not to tell. The converse of *passing* is *telling*. Several of the women reported this urge to tell, to gain sympathy for their distress and to gain praise for how they were coping with it. Sometimes this urge to tell led the women to mention this operation at unexpected times. They found that this form of self-disclosure was often mirrored as their companion shared a crisis they had recently experienced. Her account emphasized the positive features of disclosure. She scorned those who advised her to keep silent. She argued: 'I approve of telling people. It's good for the teller and the tellee. Why should humans hide their misfortunes from other humans, who are also vulnerable?'

An alternative account of the experience of breast cancer is that provided by the French writer Annie Ernaux (Ernaux & Marie, 2024). She detailed how she managed her chemotherapy while at the same time enjoying an intense love affair. She recalled the prayer of Blaise Pascal that was recited in her childhood: 'Prayer to Ask of God the Proper Use of Sickness'. Ernaux added: 'It seems to me I have made the best possible use of cancer' (p. 72). Here, she was transforming cancer from something to be endured into something that she could use. She later wrote that she detested novels or films with fictional characters who have cancer. These portrayals, she felt, were so fake. She had replaced any fear and anxiety about the disease with the excitement of an intense love affair. These novels and autobiographies contribute to a fearsome image of cancer, which is reflected in the studies of social representations of the disease.

6.2.2 *Cancer in 1980s Northern Ireland*

Fear of cancer: In the study described in the previous chapter, in which a sample of women in Northern Ireland was interviewed about health and illness, we also asked them specifically about their views on cancer. This was accompanied by a survey of 365 men and 389 women (Murray & McMillan, 1993). This survey confirmed that cancer was the most feared disease, especially among women (Table 6.1).

Thematic analysis of the interview transcripts identified five main reasons for fear of the disease: (a) *perceived incurability*, (b) *pain and suffering*, (c) *impact on family*, (d) *hereditary nature* and (e) *more common*. The major reason given for fearing cancer more than other diseases was that it was perceived as being *incurable*. For example, one woman said: 'Well, some people believe there is a cure, but I don't believe it. People will come out and say, "Oh, she's cured", you know, but I don't believe that anybody has been cured of cancer'. The possibility of it *recurring* was another aspect of this fear, e.g., 'Even if you had a bit of it removed, there's always the fear that it will come back'.

The second reason for the fear was the perceived *pain and suffering* associated with cancer, particularly among those women who had witnessed relatives dying from the disease, e.g., 'Because I watched my mother suffer with it and die with it ... it's a slow torture, you know'. This fear was part of the concern about the *type of death*.

Another concern was the *impact on the family* and what would happen to their children if they had cancer, e.g., 'It's not even the pain, but just lying knowing that you're going to die and leave the children behind'.

Table 6.1 Most frightening diseases

	Male	*Female*	*Chi-square*
Cancer	49.9%	58.3%	4.9*
Heart disease	22.0%	8.2%	25.37***
Mental illness	10.4%	16.3%	5.18*
AIDS	11.9%	10.8%	0.20
Bronchitis	0.6%	0.5%	0.00
Several	5.3%	5.8%	0.08
N	337	343	

Source Murray and McMillan (1993). Significance of male/female difference $^{*}p < 0.05$; $^{***}p < 0.001$

This concern about the impact on the family was an extension of the *illness-as-family-disruption* described in the previous chapter.

The fourth concern was the suspicion that cancer was *hereditary* since their mothers had died from it. A few women also mentioned that their fear was based on their experience of, at one time, thinking they had cancer themselves. As one woman explained: 'I have a terrible fear of cancer, mainly because last year I thought I had it myself. I had a lump removed from my breast, but of course I thought the worst ... but they removed it and it was okay. But I just have this fear of cancer'.

Several respondents feared cancer more because of their belief that cancer is becoming *more common*, particularly breast and cervical cancer. The following extract exemplifies this concern:

> For some reason I just always have it in the back of my mind, you know, cancer... especially if you're a woman. They're inclined to take it more, aren't they? You know, cancer of the womb and breast and everything. Well, that would be my main worry.

One woman explained that her fear of cancer had once been so great that she had been forced to seek counselling, which had now resolved her fear of dying.

Cancer was equated with death by the majority of women, although different aspects of dying from cancer were salient to different participants. However, it was not just any death, but one involving pain and suffering, and the prolonged nature of a cancer-related death was also emphasized.

Character of cancer: The women's descriptions of cancer in the interviews were coded into four categories: *eating-away disease, incurable nature, biomedical* and *umbrella term*. The most common description was of cancer as an *eating-away disease*. As one participant said:

> 'It just eats up your whole system doesn't it ... once it sets in, it sort of goes through you'. Another added. 'It's like something eating you inside, you know. It is just eating and eating away and leaving you with nothing'.

In this sense, the women conceived of cancer almost as a malevolent little beast destroying the body from within. They were ontologizing the disease (Herzlich and Pierret, 1987), giving it a sense of independent being. This characterization also connected with something that seems to be a widespread source of fear—little animals. Arrindell et al. (1991) reviewed

38 studies of self-assessed fears conducted in different countries. They identified fear of small animals as one of the four major classes of fear (the others being interpersonal events; death, injuries, illness, blood and surgical procedures; and agoraphobia). In normal circumstances, this fear can be controlled by taking avoidant action against the small animal. However, in the case of cancer, the malevolent being is within the individual and cannot be avoided.

The second most popular theme defined cancer with reference to its *incurable nature*. As one woman said: 'It's a disease that just can't be cured ... that's the most terrifying part about it, that there is no cure for it, you know'. Two women described cancer as 'the worst thing that could happen to a woman' on account of perhaps having to have her breast or womb removed. One woman said: 'It's a dreaded word for me'. Another added: 'It's a word I hate mentioning ... it's a subject I don't like talking about'. The third category was the *biomedical* and included such comments as: 'It's cells inside you ... one takes over the other', or 'I know cancer is abnormal cells that take over other cells'. Others regarded the word 'cancer' as an *umbrella term* for a number of different diseases.

The terms used by the women in the interviews to describe cancer were included in the survey questionnaire, which confirmed the popularity of the 'eating away' description (Table 6.2). The women were also likely to describe it in terms of a long, lingering disease and as a dreaded word.

Taken together, it would suggest that the women *objectified* cancer as something alien to themselves in terms of rotting, death and cells—contrasting views of the anthropomorphic and the biomedical. The anthropomorphic view of something rotting connects with the widespread perception of disgust. Herzlich and Pierret (1987) noted that notions of decay and putrefaction have historically dominated descriptions of internal bodily ills. However, unlike leprosy, which is visible on the body of the afflicted, the rottenness of cancer is concealed. It is this concealed nature of the decay that adds to the disgust. Disgust is associated with feelings of revulsion and nausea, fear of contagion and avoidance of disgusting objects (Davey, 2011). The impact of this on people diagnosed with cancer was a certain disgust towards their own body. This aspect would heighten the othering of the person with cancer as a means of protecting oneself from possible contagion.

In the early 1980s, Balshem (1990) conducted interviews about cancer with female residents of a working-class community in Philadelphia. She found that they had a similar anthropomorphic view

Table 6.2 Terms used to describe cancer

	Male	*Female*	*Chi-square*
An eating-away disease	34.1%	24.8%	7.3**
Abnormal cells	17.6%	20.9%	1.18
A death sentence	18.2%	17.8%	0.02
A long, lingering disease	13.2%	17.8%	2.80**
An umbrella term	11.5%	4.2%	13.03***
A dreaded word	3.8%	9.5%	8.88**
Worst thing for a woman	0.6%	4.25%	9.48
Several	0.9%	0.8%	0.00
N	340	359	

Source Murray and McMillan (1993). Significance of male/female difference $^{**}p < 0.01$, $^{***}p < 0.001$

of the disease: it was a hidden evil. One woman described cancer as a 'big black thing':

> Oh, God, I have this terrible thought of cancer – it's like a great big thing that's eating up your whole insides. This big black thing. I just think of it as black. This big black thing that just goes along like a pacman gobbling up your insides ... The movie *The Blob*, remember the blob would eat stuff and kept getting bigger. Well, that's kind of how I think of cancer. This great big blob of stuff that keeps increasing (p. 158).

Causes of cancer: The descriptions of cancer were connected with the perceived causes of the disease. In general, there was a great deal of *uncertainty* concerning the causes of cancer. As one woman stated: 'I mean the causes of the disease are just opinions really... But with the exception of smoking and, say, things like asbestos, things like that which have been almost proved.'

Despite this uncertainty, the women did suggest a range of possible causes of cancer. These were grouped into five main categories: *Environment, Biomedical, Heredity, Lifestyle* and *Stress and Worry. Environmental factors* included air pollution, microwave ovens, asbestos, working conditions, and nuclear radiation. As one woman said: 'Well, it certainly isn't doing us any good. I think a lot more investigation should go into towns where there is a chemical factory for it gives off an awful lot of toxic fumes'.

The second category was *Biomedical factors,* which included X-rays and the overuse of antibiotics, e.g.,

> I think if you go and get an antibiotic every time you come up against a minor infection, that when you come up against something, the body stops fighting of its own accord. It could be one of the causes of cancer, if people use something artificial to fight off every minor illness ... As well as that people are only using them relatively recently so that nobody knows what effect using antibiotics for 20 or 30 years would have. It could cause the body to develop a cancer.

The third cause was *heredity,* which referred to some intrinsic characteristic of the individual that naturally developed into cancer or was provoked by a rather insignificant event, such as a fall. For example, one woman said:

> I don't think the environment has anything to do with it. I'm a firm believer in if a thing's there, it's going to come out anyway eventually. If it's in your system, it will come out sooner or later.

The fourth category was *lifestyle and attitude*, which included smoking and diet as potential causes. For example:

> I think that everybody is a potential cancer victim but I think if they try and keep their general health up to a certain level by eating reasonably well ... I would imagine that would help to prevent cancer.

It also included the general attitude of the person.

A fifth factor was *stress and worry.* It was felt that this was especially the case among women, e.g., 'Well, I don't know, but I think women have a lot more on their plate with worry and what have you... I do think worry can bring it on sometimes.'

These descriptions of cancer could be grouped into two larger categories: (1) *exogenous*—environment, biomedical, modern world and genetics; (2) *endogenous*—lifestyle and attitude. There was a tension between these two categories. On the one hand, by othering the source of cancer in the environment and the modern world, the person could protect themselves from blame. However, it was not straightforward, for it also depended on the person's lifestyle, including smoking, diet and general attitude. While initially, some people could then be held responsible for developing cancer, this was not the case for these working-class women who had to face the stress of modern life.

These descriptions of the causes of cancer were a means of *anchoring* the disease in the modern world. These causes were phenomena over which they had little control and were features of modern society. In the same way that Herzlich (1973) talked about the impact of modern society, one woman said: ‘Too many people have broken away from the old-fashioned—living—you know’. The modern world was talked about in terms of environmental hazards, stress and food additives. One woman said:

> I think I read somewhere once that sometimes people after a divorce or after a death seem to develop cancer, and I think it depends on the way they cope with it - some people can cope with these - things - and some people just cannot cope with these things. I think if you’re a kind of positive person or a reasonably optimistic person, that maybe helps to prevent cancer.

These working-class women thought that they were more at risk of cancer for both biomedical and social reasons. The explanations given for women’s greater susceptibility to cancer were related mainly to *biological* differences between men and women. Several women suggested that childbirth itself might be a factor in women’s greater vulnerability:

> I think mostly women take cancer ... because of the different parts of their body ... they go through so many changes. Even having a baby your body changes ... different things like that. I think that’s the reason why they do take it more than men.

A further explanation given for women’s greater susceptibility was that women have more *stressful lives*. Two women suggested that women are inclined to *pay less attention to themselves*:

> I mean women have a fear... you know they’re aware of the risks of cancer because there are smear tests and all available, and yet they go along saying, ‘I’m alright... it won’t happen to me... I’ve too much to do to be worrying about my health’. I would say she doesn’t take as much time in looking after herself.

These negative social representations of the disease as something disgusting, which could possibly reflect on the moral character of the person afflicted, were commonplace. For this reason, the women with breast cancer often attempted to conceal the disease. However, the women were reluctant to take responsibility for the disease. It was something largely outside their control.

6.2.3 Cancer in 2010s Palestine

The West Bank is the area of Palestine to the west of the River Jordan. Since the establishment of this region, the Palestinian residents have experienced sustained oppression by Israeli settlers and the Israeli Defence Force. Everyday life for the Palestinians there has been one of constant harassment and displacement (Amnesty International, 2024a). Between 2008 and 2024, over 7000 Palestinian civilian residents in the West Bank were killed and over 150,000 injured as a direct result of the occupation and conflict (UNOCHA, 2025). The vicious repression experienced by the Palestinian residents of the West Bank was graphically displayed in the television documentary by Theroux (2025) and recent evidence indicates that Israeli settlers are intensifying their efforts to drive out Palestinians (Bowen, 2025). The wholescale oppression of the Palestinian people has intensified with the Israeli government's ongoing genocide in Gaza which has led to the death of tens of thousands of Palestinians in that region (Amnesty International, 2024b; Shlaim, 2024; UNOCHA, 2025). Despite this, the Palestinian administration has organized a health service and taken steps to manage the most serious health problems. In the early 2000s, similar to the Western countries, the major causes of death identified were heart disease and cancer.

As in other societies, cancer is socially enmeshed in the social representations of the disease held by the residents of Palestine. In a study conducted in 2013 (Albarghouthi & Klempe, 2019), a sample of 16 male and female residents was interviewed about the disease. All the interviews were conducted in Arabic, and the transcriptions were subjected to thematic analysis, beginning with an inductive approach and then linking the themes together using a deductive approach.

Four main themes were constructed from their descriptions of cancer: (a) *vagueness and ambiguity*, (b) *proximity to death*, (c) *metaphorical character* of cancer and (d) *social re-presentations of cancer*. The *vagueness and ambiguity* theme concerned the difficulty of grasping the character of the disease. Often, participants felt it was difficult to talk about it, e.g., 'I do not think that I will be useful in this talk, I do not know much about this disease'. It was suggested that this reluctance to talk about the disease might reflect the Arabic socio-cultural context, where there is a hesitation to discuss illness and death. Instead, there is the use of various euphemisms and the invocation of religious protectors, e.g., 'Allhom A'fena' ('May God protect and give us health'). It might also reflect, to a certain extent, a form of self-protection from the potential threat posed by the disease.

A related theme was the *association with death*. As one participant said: 'It is accumulated in the Palestinian consciousness that that disease leads to death'. Here, the use of the term 'that disease' rather than 'cancer' reflected the anxiety about the disease. In addition, the reference to 'Palestinian consciousness' was an indicator of the historical and socio-cultural dimension. As Wagoner (2015) asserted: 'Social representations are carriers of collective memory, through them past experiences shape the present'.

The *metaphorical character* of cancer refers to the use of metaphors for cancer to avoid referring directly to it while also expanding the character of the disease. Metaphors for cancer often take the form of euphemisms, including various Arabic terms such as 'Al-Khabith' ('the malignant cunning disease') or 'Al Marad Al-A'atel' ('the bad/nasty disease'). These euphemisms reflect the Arabic belief that words can impact people's lives. There is also the use of military metaphors such as 'invasion' and 'colonize', which reflect the everyday experience of the Palestinian people who have been under occupation for 50 years. These military metaphors are also present in descriptions of cancer treatment.

The final theme introduced more *positive images* of cancer. These centred on improvements in treatment and the value of early detection. As one participant said: 'People think if you have cancer, you will die. That is not true' (p. 114). This *re-presentation of cancer* was particularly prominent among the younger, more educated participants.

There were certain paradoxical social representations of cancer. These included *pity-based societal responses* such as paradoxical displays of sympathy, empathy, compassion and stigma. Although the patient was pitied, s/he could also be 'othered' as a victim of a dreadful disease. In turn, the patient could internalize these reactions through self-pity and self-stigma. The patient might attempt to manage this by avoiding telling others about the disease.

The second aspect of paradoxical representations of cancer was in the *manifestations of stigma*. Here, the patient was perceived as vulnerable, as if they were dying and demanding care. But at the same time, the patient was expected to show courage and bravery and to fight back against the disease. The social stigma of cancer meant that people were embarrassed about the diagnosis and its impact on the family in a conservative society. It was suggested that this reflected broader cultural and religious values. One participant described the impact on the family: 'Yes, she was even terrified about affecting the marriage chances of her daughters and grand-daughters more than her own health'.

The third paradoxical theme was *cancer rumours*. The negative outlook for cancer patients fuelled the growth of rumours about a person's life chances. An example of the role of rumours was the comment by one participant: 'You know, people gather and start talking: oh, have you heard about our neighbor, oh poor her, they say she got the malignant disease, she is still young and has small children'. However, there was also evidence that times were changing and that people were more optimistic, and the negative rumours were less impactful. As a result, the 'othering' of the cancer person was more restrained. As one participant recalled: 'People hesitated to visit my father because they thought that cancer was contagious'.

Another major feature was the *religious discourse*. This had three sub-themes: cancer as predestined by the *will of God*, cancer as a *punishment* or a trial, and cancer as a *spiritual journey* of healing. Each of these sub-themes emphasized the strength of religion in the Palestinian community. Cancer was governed by God's laws; it was part of God's plan, it was evidence of God's displeasure, and it was an opportunity for the person to embark on a spiritual journey.

This study illustrated the cognitive polyphasia, or the different and contradictory knowledge systems held by these Palestinians. These were a mixture of biomedical, sociocultural, religious and political frames. It emphasized the changing cultural and religious context within which people developed an understanding of the disease. The most common explanation was in terms of an 'invasion' from some threatening source, which 'colonized' the body and could be treated by some 'counter-attack'. These military metaphors all highlighted the political context of the Palestinian people, as they compared cancer with the Israeli occupation of their land and illustrated how large political processes can pervade everyday social representations.

6.3 Mental Illness

There has been a steady increase in the fear of mental illness across the world. According to the IPSOS (2024) survey, it has replaced cancer as the most feared health issue. This is followed by stress, obesity and drug abuse. This fear of mental illness is especially prominent among women.

6.3.1 Artistic Images of Mental Illness

Mental illness has been a frequent theme in art, literature and films. The 'madman' is often depicted as someone who does not conform to social norms. For example, the Greek god Dionysus was not only the god of wine and pleasure but also of madness and frenzy. He was also represented as withdrawn or hermitic and as someone with strange physical properties and abilities. Scull (2015) detailed how madness has been represented in art throughout the ages. In ancient biblical texts, there were accounts of madness due to devil possession or divine displeasure. This religious imagery was also balanced with more naturalistic approaches, which developed into biomedical models. However, ancient ideas about mental illness continue to persist.

Foucault (1965), in his historical analysis *Madness and Civilization*, described the changing social attitudes towards mental illness in Western society. In the Renaissance, the madman was represented in art as someone who possessed a certain kind of wisdom about the world. With the rise of industrial capitalism, people with mental illness were no longer accepted and were instead perceived as a threat to society, leading to their confinement in large institutions. Artistic portrayals often situated them in such places. Moscovici ([1976] 2008) referred to this work, noting that 'determining the boundaries between the normal and the pathological is one of society's most important tasks' (p. 72).

In the modern era, people with mental illness often feature in films. Six main stereotypes of such portrayals were identified by Hyler (1988): (a) the *homicidal maniac*, (b) the *rebellious free spirit*, (c) the *enlightened member of society*, (d) the *female patient as seductress*, (e) the *narcissistic parasite* and (f) the *zoo specimen*. A more recent review noted the continuation of these negative images and added two more types: the *simpleton* and the *victim* (Pirkis et al., 2006). Perhaps the most famous film portrayal of mental illness in film was *One Flew Over the Cuckoo's Nest*

(1975), which was based on the same-titled novel by Ken Kesey. Although the film was a comedy, it portrayed the characters from a mental institution as strange and unpredictable.

In the 1980s, and again 30 years later, de Rosa conducted a series of studies on social representations of madness (de Rosa, 1987, De Rosa & Bocca, 2018). She asked a sample of children and adults to describe in words and to draw a picture of a mad person. The younger children's words and pictures emphasized deviance and identified prisons as the most suitable therapeutic regime. The older children used more medicalized representations of madness and identified the importance of medical doctors as those concerned with therapeutic treatment. The adolescents' and adults' representations were more psychological rather than physical and identified psychologists and psychiatrists as the therapeutic agents.

In an analysis of the drawings, de Rosa identified three primary images of the madman: magical-fantastic (monsters and demons), deviant (criminal, drug addict) and medical (physically handicapped, mentally ill). The magical-fantastic drawings portrayed both positive and negative images of the madman, reflecting the twofold face of madness in history. On the one hand, there was the jester who exhibited expressive and creative freedom, while, on the other, there was the monster who exhibited malignant supernatural forces. There were also drawings of the madman as an artist or a boffin/genius. The deviant images included drawings of prisoners and drunks, while the medical images depicted people with various physical deformities.

In analysing the pictures, de Rosa noted the presence of classic stigmatizing features of madness, such as staring eyes and horns. She argued that these images could be traced to medieval depictions of madness, indicating cultural-historical influences on the children's representations. There was evidence of cognitive polyphasia, with archaic representations of madness mingling with more modern representations. While the more modern representations may contribute to inclusion, the more archaic representations contribute to exclusion. Compared with the images collected in the 1980s, the later drawings presented more medicalized images, indicating the growing dominance of medical discourse about mental illness.

6.3.2 Mental Illness in 1970s France

The classic study of social representations of mental illness was conducted by Denise Jodelet in France in the early 1970s, although it was not published until much later (Jodelet, 1989/1991). This study was conducted during the period of de-institutionalization of residents from long-term psychiatric facilities. Various initiatives in the form of community care for people with mental health problems were being explored. Jodelet's study was a detailed investigation of a village in France that, for over a 100 years, had been providing accommodation and support for people with various mental health problems. The villagers, who called themselves the *civilians*, provided lodging for the mentally ill, who were referred to as the *bredins*, or the loonies. These individuals worked in a large facility on the edge of the village.

This intensive ethnographic study used a variety of methods to explore the social representations of mental illness among the villagers. Lasting four years, it was the archetypal socio-cultural study of social representations. Its aim was to 'identify at all levels of social life the forms which the relationship with insanity assumes, the conditions for its acceptance, and the representations associated with it' (p. 17). There were five main phases to the study:

1. Observation of everyday activities through engagement in community life.
2. Reconstruction of the history through analysis of relevant literature and interviews with key personnel.
3. Description of the organization of family placement through interviews with medical staff.
4. Description of the details of the placements and foster parents through a survey of the placement families and patients.
5. Description of how the community positioned itself regarding the lodgers through detailed interviews with foster parents.

The wealth of information collected from these different sources was then systematically reviewed and integrated into a detailed account of the organization of the community. The approach also identified certain surprising features of community life, such as water being reserved by the residents for personal use and the treatment of items touched by the lodgers.

Theoretically, Jodelet defined social representations as 'a form of social thought whose genesis, properties and functions have to be viewed in relation to the processes which affect social life and communication, the mechanisms which tend towards the definition of the identity and specificity of social subjects, individuals or groups, as well as the energies which underlie the relationships formed by those with one another' (p. 15). Thus, the aim was not simply to describe residents' symbolic representations of the mentally ill, but how they interacted with them in their everyday lives.

A key issue was the 'othering' of the lodgers. The civilians/foster parents tended to isolate themselves from them, which led to some unusual practices, some of which were promoted by the medical authorities. For example, the foster parents were required to install a window in their living rooms so that they could keep an eye on the lodgers, who resided in a separate part of the house. This separation into different rooms reflected a certain fear about the presence of the lodger in the house.

Looking through the historical medical records, Jodelet noted that when the scheme started, the residents were very anxious about the patients. For example, one record noted: 'They were thought to be unmanageable, violent, even dangerous'. But over time, especially through careful selection of patients by the medical doctors, the residents became more accepting, e.g., 'And so we heard people say: "For madmen, they are very quiet"; "You would think they were quite middle class"' (p. 35). However, there remained a hidden anxiety, which was exhibited through the residents' interactions with the patients. At the same time, the residents were keen to present their community to outsiders as 'normal' by characterizing certain actions of lodgers as a normal part of everyday life.

In their everyday lives, the lodgers, the 'non-civilians', were treated as different. In the family home, the lodger had separate meals from the rest of the family and did not participate in family leisure activities. Although they treated them as different, the foster parents were reluctant to talk about them as having a mental illness. 'The embarrassment and reticence shown by our interviewees at directly confronting in conversation any aspect of the lodger's psychiatric state was shown in their statements, their hesitations, their refusals, their silences, their evasion or recasting of questions, physical signs of discomfort (blushing, sweating, trembling of the hands, laughter, etc.)' (p. 149). It was only through close observation of their interactions that an understanding of their social representations of mental illness was developed.

The lodgers were different but also, in many ways, the same. 'The inability to act for themselves has repercussions for the social life of the patients, not just in their modes of participation as productive, responsible agents within the community, but also in the forms of socialization and, it might be said, sociability, that are mentality and morality' (p. 187). Their ability to work seemed to make the lodgers similar to the residents. Work organized their day and gave them an opportunity for wider social interaction, just as it did for the residents.

The foster parents distinguished between those lodgers whose mental illness was more organic than social: 'It all depends on the type of illness he's got, whether he's a nervous case, or whether he's subnormal' (p. 199). Different names were used to characterize different lodgers, ranging from the 'crackpot' to the 'nutter' to the 'head case'. Each had particular types of mental illness. The degree of anxiety depended upon the type of patient. The most feared was the patient with epilepsy. The foster parents would say that they were anxious because an epileptic fit would frighten their children. Details of a fit were recounted, referring to gestures of brutality and sexuality. Then there was the dribble and foaming around the mouth during a fit, which raised fears of contagion. Jodelet summarized this fear:

> If foam, the slaver of an overheated, excited or rabid animal, recalls an instinctive and bestial element in human make-up which resides in uncontrolled strength, violence and sexuality, then the association of nerves and organic fluids, whose interaction marks phases of excitation, is also confirmed (p. 227).

Despite assurances from the medical authorities, there was the fear of contagion. The foster parents could protect themselves by distancing but also by not talking about it. 'A resurgence of the illness is prevented by avoiding any reference to it when speaking with those who live in its shadows. This absolute refusal to speak of it wards off the alarming possibility of its appearance' (p. 232). The process of objectification of the illness in the brain of the patient was not sufficient to ward off the anxiety rooted in ancient beliefs. Medication was important as it implied an organic basis for the illness. The absence of medication meant the illness was due to moral innocence or wickedness. The former was deserving of acceptance, and the latter of punishment of some sort.

The foster parents found it difficult to explain why they treated the patients differently. Instead, they simply emphasized that it was the usual way or a custom. For example, in the case of the household eating routine, one woman said:

> I take them their meals, it's me who collects their dishes. I do my washing-up and everything. I don't like anyone touching. That's something I insist on ... I don't let them touch things which belong to the house. No, no, no. I do my washing up first and then I do theirs ... I don't know why ... It's a habit of mine (p. 242).

This behaviour reflected a hidden social representation:

> The representation which guides it is hidden somewhere in the concern for hygiene and the contradictory evocation of a denied contagion. It is a mute thought whose attendant actions designate its true belief: the transmissibility of insanity (p. 243).

Jodelet suggested that the avoidance of touching the patient's fluids was a 'materialized' representation of the illness. Protecting the children was often used as a reason for separating the washing. Separate eating utensils were used.

In conclusion, Jodelet commented on the multiple factors that explained the representations of the foster parents. She termed this 'the problem of multiple symbolism, of the polysemy of interdiction, of the over-determination of the behaviour' (p. 264). To clarify these processes, she introduced Mauss's (1950) idea of poles of magic and religion. The three properties of magic are protection against certain properties of the patients, the secret, intimate way in which patients are kept and the individual variability of rule-keeping. Religion promoted certain moral laws about behaviour that aimed at respect for the family circle. These two poles or dimensions summarized how the foster parents managed the patients.

Jodelet concluded by describing social representations of mental illness as composed of different constituents derived from various sources, including direct relationships with practice, the community's values and lifestyle, the community's local culture and traditional knowledge and the medical knowledge obtained from conversations with health staff. These representations 'take on the form of a fluid, fuzzy, and not intangible, reservoir whose actualizations vary with context and use' (p. 289). Thus, the social representations of mental illness in the community were not fixed but depended upon the individual concerned and the immediate social context.

In their discussion of the narrative content of social representations of history, Liu and László (2007) refer to two key properties of narratives—perspective-taking and empathy generation. Applying such an approach to Jodelet's study, it was apparent that their social representations provided a certain perspective on the mentally ill patients. In addition, it could generate a certain empathy not just for the mentally ill but also for the foster parents. On the one hand, the patients were attempting to be considered normal by going to work and fulfilling certain everyday tasks, while the foster parents were helping those who were experiencing mental health challenges by providing food and accommodation.

6.3.3 Mental Illness in 1990s Britain and France

It would be expected that health professionals would be more likely to have a medicalized view of mental illness. However, several studies have confirmed that the picture is much more complex, reflecting the changing character of care for the mentally ill.

During the 1990s, a study by Morant (1995) found that this was not clear-cut. She interviewed 30 mental health professionals in London and a similar number in Paris. Analysis of the interview transcripts revealed a high degree of uncertainty about the nature of mental illness. Three main themes—difference, disruption and distress—were used to describe mental illness. Difference concerned the quantitative difference in the cases of neurosis and the qualitative difference in the case of psychosis, as well as whether all forms of mental illness are simply exaggerations of normal experience. Disruption concerned the extent of disturbance to personal and social life. Distress revolved around the fear, feelings of loss of control and hopelessness felt by people with mental illness.

The professionals worked in multidisciplinary teams, which had less focus on the body or mind (classic medical approach) and more on improving the person's personal and social life. The turn to more community-based care would seem to have augmented uncertainties in their representations. It was felt that the traditional dominance of psychiatry had been challenged by multidisciplinary teamwork. There were certain differences between the British and the French, with the French view reflecting more strongly the influence of the psychodynamic approach.

It was suggested that the uncertainty in the representations of the mental health professionals reflected the changing policy context and the shift to community care. While there were echoes of the expert knowledge systems, these were modulated with attention to the main representational themes. Also, differences in the conceptual models were ignored as the health professionals adopted a bricoleur approach, incorporating both biomedical and more social approaches. Finally, there was less evidence of the clear-cut othering of the mental patient; instead, the health professionals represented mental illness in a more ambiguous way that was less unanimously rejecting.

Theoretically, this study showed that these professionals' representations drew upon both reified and consensual knowledge systems (see Chap. 3). There was also evidence of the importance of the power dynamic within these representations, indicating that the policy makers driving the agenda of community care had a disproportionate influence. The traditional power of the medical profession is being challenged, but the voice of the mentally ill client remains underdeveloped.

6.3.4 *Mental Illness in 2010s Canada*

In a study conducted by Negura et al. (2020) in Canada a sample of adults who had experienced or were experiencing depression completed a word-association task about depression, followed by a semi-structured interview. In addition, the team conducted an analysis of newspaper articles about depression. Both sets of data were then subjected to a lexicographic analysis and a more qualitative analysis to explore the underlying social representations. They were particularly interested in the power dynamics within the social representations of depression.

They considered the social representations of depression as operating at the three different levels suggested by Jodelet (2012). At the trans-subjective level, the 'medical expertise is associated with a competence that is reserved for physicians and emanates from scientific knowledge, whose representation is itself anchored in the sacred/profane thema' (p. 7). This sacred/profane thema is an ancient dichotomy that confers legitimacy upon certain social representations. As Negura et al. continue: 'What puts a physician in the initiated class is not only a consequence of his coolly and rationally applied knowledge and expertise, but is also owed to a particular status that has been granted and consecrated to him' (p. 7). Thus, the physician is granted a priest-like status, drawing upon their socio-cultural heritage. This anchoring of medical knowledge gives the physician legitimacy regarding their actions and biological interpretation of depression. This biological interpretation of depression is strongly related to the sacred/profane thema and gives the medical treatment legitimacy.

At the inter-subjective level, these social representations of depression intervene in our social interaction. The medical representation is the dominant or hegemonic representation, which imposes itself on the management of depression. However, there is also a social representation of depression that emphasizes the role of traumatic experiences, although they do not directly oppose the medical representation. In their study of newspapers, Negura et al. also identified a more polemic representation of depression, which explained it with reference to modern society and the potential value of a simpler life as the appropriate management strategy. This polemic representation directly challenges the hegemonic medical representation but also connects with the recurring 'way of life' representation of illness.

At the subjective level, the person with depression internalizes the power relations of the medical representation. The participants explained depression as 'an invisible handicap, that is, as an inability to respond to social expectations regarding how to function in society according to normalized roles—a handicap that is not recognized or understood as such by family and friends' (pp. 12–13). As such, the person with depression was defined in medical terms, requiring medical treatment. This showed the dominance of the biomedical approach.

6.4 Anchoring and Othering

There were certain common features in the social representations of these diseases, both ancient and modern. A paramount factor is the anchoring of the genesis of the disease in the 'other'. This was often followed by the exclusion or isolation of those with the disease. This process of othering reflected the broader tensions in society at particular times and places.

In the case of HIV/AIDS, this othering was associated with the supposed aberrant sexual practices of certain minority groups. In Britain, gay men were initially the target of a moralizing discourse at the outbreak of the AIDS epidemic. This was at a time when there was increasing debate about gay rights and the introduction of legislation to decriminalize homosexual acts. In Africa, the moralizing discourse regarding HIV/AIDS remained strong in those countries with a strong Protestant tradition, while it declined in others.

In the case of COVID-19, the initial othering was of the Chinese, especially their food handling practices. This occurred at a time when there was political anxiety in the West over the increasing power of China and evidence of heightened xenophobia towards Chinese immigrants. In the case of cancer, the cause of the disease was perceived as stemming from various exogenous factors, including the environment and way of life. This was at a time when there was increasing debate about climate change. Similarly, the rise in mental illness was attributed to the stresses of modern life during a period of rapid technological and social change.

This process of anchoring the cause of the disease in the other spread to the 'othering' of the person afflicted. Although these people may not be the ultimate source of the health problem, as carriers, they could possibly spread the disease to others. This fear of physical contagion was associated with the ancient fear of the contagion of infectious diseases. It was felt that people with these health problems needed to be kept at a distance, although the degree of distance depended upon the extent to which it was felt to be controllable. People with low social status and those from foreign lands who adopted different eating practices were particularly the target of this othering.

This othering leads to stigmatization, discrimination, and exclusion from valued activities. The internalization of this negative social representation leads to various self-protection strategies. The most common is the concealment of the health problem or potentially recasting it as something valuable. People who have a health problem can conceal it and pass as normal, or disclose it with apprehension about the reaction of their companions.

Another component of the social representation of the health problem was the extent to which the person is responsible for it and the extent to which he or she challenges it. Diseases were often attributed to exogenous factors over which the person had little control. In the cancer stories, it was emphasized by the women that they did not deserve to have the disease. However, they did attempt to control it, to fight against the disease. The good patient was the one who did not accept the disease but struggled to overcome it. This was the illness-as-occupation described by Herzlich (1973). The struggle could be in conjunction with both medicine and religion. Such a fightback could be at an individual level, but it could also be at a societal level, as in the case of the so-called war against cancer and other diseases. However, in the case of the 'spoiled identity', there was a certain acceptance that the afflicted person had a degree of responsibility.

Another aspect of the social representation of several diseases was the silence it engendered. This was especially the case with women's social representation of cancer. The disease was to be feared, and to talk about it raised the possibility of attracting it: 'let sleeping dogs lie'. Contemporary diseases are often surrounded by social representations that convey fear and anxiety. These fears draw upon historical, artistic, and media representations of different diseases. These representations seem to have been adopted for certain illnesses from an early age. Cancer was the contemporary major fear because of its frequency, supposed incurability and associated pain and suffering. For women, there was also the concern about the impact on the family. Women particularly feared breast cancer.

Social representations are reflected in our culture and everyday practices. We may avoid situations where contact with people who have certain diseases occurs without being conscious of our behaviour. Our lowered tone of voice when discussing someone who has developed a particular disease reflects a certain anxiety about it. The confinement of diseased individuals to institutions, especially isolated institutions, adds to the negative social representations.

Social representations of particular diseases have implications for our everyday social interactions and for the identity of the person impacted. Not only does it lead to the person with the disease being avoided, but the person impacted also develops strategies to avoid this exclusion. They can achieve this by concealing the diagnosis of the disease and attempting to pass as normal. They can also attempt to challenge a stigmatizing representation and present a more positive representation, but this is difficult on an individual level.

With the growth of biomedicine, there was increasing confidence in its ability to control disease. However, the emergence of new infectious diseases seemed to challenge this optimistic viewpoint. There is a certain suspicion about medicine, particularly regarding the role of the pharmaceutical industry. This became especially pronounced in the case of COVID-19. Priniski and Holyoak (2022) found that a certain scepticism about the credibility of medical science and a suspicion regarding the promotion of vaccines had developed. Conspiracy theories have historically emerged in society during times of social uncertainty. Modern conspiracy culture has been traced back to the aftermath of the French Revolution, where it was associated with secret societies such as the Freemasons (Byford, 2011). During periods of uncertainty, conspiracy theories can provide a simple explanation and a means of taking action (van Prooijen & Douglas, 2017). This seems to be the case for new diseases such as COVID-19, where attention focused on the role of the pharmaceutical industry. In the case of cancer, there was more generalized reference to the modern way of life as a cause of the disease, but also to environmental factors such as the nuclear and pharmaceutical industries. Together, these examples indicate how social representations of diseases are connected to historical changes in society. This aligns with evidence of a certain apprehension, especially among people from lower socio-economic backgrounds, about medical and pharmaceutical advances (Binsemael et al., 2024). New diseases will emerge and social representation theory can help explore how people begin to make sense of them often drawing upon ancient as well as contemporary experiences.

References

Albarghouthi, S. I., & Klempe, S. H. (2019). "Al-Khabith"—The malignant cunning disease. Socio-cultural complexity and social representations of cancer in the occupied Palestine territory. *Journal of Health Psychology*, *25*(1), 99–131.

Alpert, J. S. (2024). Leprosy in literature and art: The covenant of water. *American Journal of Medicine*, *137*(7), 559–560.

Amnesty International. (2024a). Spike in Israeli Lethal Force against Palestinians in occupied West Bank.

Amnesty International. (2024b). 'You feel like you are subhuman'. Israel's genocide against Palestinians in Gaza. *Amnesty International.*

Arnold-Foster, A. (2021). *The cancer problem: Malignancy in nineteenth-century Britain.* Oxford University Press.

Arrindell, W. A., Pickersgill, M. J., Merkelbach, H., Ardon, A. M., & Cornet, F. C. (1991). Phobic dimensions: III factor analytic approaches to the study of common phobic fear. *Advances in Behaviour Research and Therapy*, *13*, 73–130.

Balshem, M. (1990). Cancer, control and causality: Talking about cancer in a working class community. *American Ethnologist*, *18*(1), 152–172.

BBC News. (2020). 2020 in pictures: Coronavirus in the UK *2020 in pictures: Coronavirus in the UK. BBC News*

Beres, L., Winskell, K., Neri, E. M., Mbukwen, B., & Obyerodhyambo, P. (2013). Making sense of HIV testing: Social representations in young Africans' HIV-related narratives. *Global Public Health*, *8*(8), 890–903.

Binsemael, A., Thornton, N., Horton, T., & Hardie, T. (2024). How does the public feel about health technologies and data? *The Health Foundation.*

Bowen, J. (2025).*Israel settlers intensify campaign to drive out West Bank Palestinians.* BBC News.

Byford, J. (2011). *Conspiracy theories: An introduction.* Palgrave Macmillan.

Camus, A. (1947). *The plague.* Penguin.

Clarke, J. N., & Everest, M. (2006). Cancer in the mass print media: Fear, uncertainty and the medical model. *Social Science and Medicine*, *62*(10), 2591–2600.

Comfort, G. (1992). *Dying to live.* Tyndale House.

Davey, D. C. L. (2011). Disgust: The disease-avoidance emotion and its dysfunctions. *Philosophical Transactions of the Royal Society London Section B*, *366*, 3453–3465.

de Rosa, A. S. (1987). The social representations of mental illness in children and adults. In W. Doise & S. Mocovici (Eds.), *Current issues in European social psychology* (Vol. 2, pp. 47–138). Cambridge University Press.

de Rosa, A. S., & Bocci, E. (2018). Resisting cognitive polyphasia in the social representations of madness. In A. S. de Rosa (Ed.), *Social representations in the 'Social Arena'* (pp. 245–310). Routledge.

Ernaux, A., & Marie, M. (2024). *The use of photography.* Fitzcarraldo.

Foucault, M. (1961/1965). *Madness and civilization* [*Folie et Déraison: Histoire de la Folie à l'âge classique*]. Pantheon.

Goffman, E. (1963). *Stigma. Notes on the management of spoiled identity.* Penguin.

Hajdu, S. I. (2010). A note from history: The first printed case reports of cancer. *Cancer*, *116*(10), 2493–2498.

Hawkins, A. H. (1993). *Reconstructing illness: Studies in pathography.* Purdue University Press.

Herzlich, C. (1973). *Health and illness. A social psychological analysis.* Academic Press. (Original: *Santé et Maladie: Analyse d'une Réprésentation Sociale.* Paris: Mouton, 1969).

Herzlich, C., & Pierret, J. (1980). *Illness and self in society.* Johns Hopkins University Press.

Herzlich, C., & Pierret, J. (1987). *Illness and self in society.* Johns Hopkins University Press.

Houston, A. (2016). 'Seiknes Incurabill': The evolution of literary representations of leprosy in medieval and early modern English narratives. *Chicago Journal of Medicine*, *16*, 30–41.

Hyler, S. E. (1988). DSM-III at the cinema: Madness in the movies. *Comprehensive Psychiatry*, *29*, 195–206.

Idoiaga, N., Berasategi, N., Eiguren, A., & Picaza, M. (2020). Exploring children's social and emotional representations of the COVID-19 pandemic. *Frontiers in Psychology, 11*, 1952.

IPSOS (2024). Mental health seen as the biggest health issue. In *IPSOS health service report 2024*. IPSOS.

Ittefaq, M., Abwao, M., Baines, A., Belmas, G., Kamboh, S. A., & Fiqueroa, E. J. (2022). A pandemic of hate: Social representations of COVID-19 in the media. *Analyses of Social Issues and Public Policy, 22*(1), 225–252.

Jodelet, D. (1989/1991). *Madness and social representations*. University of California Press.

Jodelet, D. (1991). *Madness and social representations. Living with the mad in one French community*. University of California Press.

Jodelet, D. (2012). Interconnections between social representations and intervention. In A. de Rosa (Ed.), *Social representations in the 'Social Arena'* (pp. 77–88). Routledge.

Joffe, H. (1996a). The shock of the new: A psychodynamic extension of social representations theory. *Journal for the Theory of Social Behaviour, 26*(2), 197–219.

Joffe, H. (1996b). AIDS research and prevention: A social representational approach. *British Journal of Medical Psychology, 69*(3), 169–190.

Joffe, H. (1999). *Risk and 'the other'*. Cambridge University Press.

Kaptein, A. A. (2021). Writing cancer. *Supportive Care in Cancer, 29*, 4375–4380.

Kaptein, A. A., Meulenberg, F., & Murray, M. (2020). Artistic representations of infectious disease. *Psychology, Health and Medicine, 25*(4), 492–496.

Kearney, A.J., & Murray, M. (2009). Breast cancer screening recommendations: Is mammography the only answer? *Journal of Midwifery & Women's Health, 54* (5), 393–400

Klein, M. (1946). Notes on some schizoid mechanisms. *International Journal of Psycho-Analysis, 27*, 99–110.

Liu, J. H., & László, J. (2007). A narrative theory of history and identity. Social identity, social representation, society, and the individual. In G. Moloney & I. Walker (Eds.), *Social representations and identity. Content, process, and power* (pp. 85–108). Palgrave.

Marková, I., & Wilkie, P. (1987). Representations, concepts and social change: The phenomenon of AIDS. *Journal for the Theory of Social Behaviour, 17*(4), 389–409.

Morant, N. (1995). What is mental illness? Social representations of mental illness. *Papers on Social Representations, 4*, 41–52.

Moscovici, S. ([1976] 2008). *Psychoanalysis: Its image and its public*. [English translation of *La psychoanalyse, son image et son image, 1976]*. Polity Press.

Murray, M. (1993). Social and cognitive representations of health and illness. In H. Schroder, K. Reschke, M. Johnson, & S. Maes (Eds.), *Health psychology—Potential in diversity* (pp. 124–131). S. Roderer Verlag.
Murray, M. (2009). Telling stories and making sense of cancer. *International Journal of Narrative Practice, 1*, 25–36.
Negura, L., Plante, N., & Lévesque, M. (2020). The role of social representations in the construction of power relations. *Journal for the Theory of Social Behaviour, 50*(1), 29–41.
Patterson, J. T. (1987). *The Dread Disease: Cancer and modern American culture*. Harvard University Press.
Pinell, P. (1987). How do cancer patients express their points of view? *Sociology of Health and Illness, 9*(1), 25–44.
Pirkis, J., Blood, R. W., Francis, C., & McMillan, K. (2006). On-screen portrayals of mental illness: Extent, nature, and impact. *Journal of Health Communication, 11* (5), 523–541.
Priniski, J. H., & Holyoak, K. J. (2022). A darkening spring: How preexisting distrust shaped COVID-19 skepticism. *PLoS One, 17*(1), 0263191.
Rabinow, P. (1986). Representations are social facts: Modernity and post-modernity in anthropology. In J. Clifford & G. E. Marcus (Eds.), *Writing culture: The poetics and politics of ethnography* (pp. 234–261). University of California Press.
Scull, A. (2015). *Madness in civilization: A history of insanity from the Bible to Freud, from the madhouse to modern medicine*. Thames & Hudson.
Shlaim, A. (2024). *Genocide in Gaza. Israel, Hamas and the long war on Palestine*. Irish Pages Press.
Sontag, S. (1977). *Illness as metaphor*. Penguin.
Souza, L. G. S., O'Dwyer, E., Coutinho, S. M., Chaudhuri, S., Rocha, L. L., & de Souza, L. P. (2021). Social representations and ideology: Theories of common-sense about COVID-19 among middle-class Brazilians and their ideological implications. *Journal of Social and Political Psychology, 9*(1), 105–122.
Theroux, L. (2025). BBC two—Louis Theroux, the settlers. Accessed 26 May 2025.
Tokarczuk, O. (2024). *The empusium. A health resort horror story*. Fitzcaraldo.
UNAIDS. (2022). *Global HIV&AIDS statistics—Fact sheet*. Geneva: UNAIDS.
UNOCHA (2025). Data on casualties|United Nations Office for the Coordination of Humanitarian Affairs—Occupied Palestinian Territory. Accessed 26 May 2025.
Vaidya, J. S. (2007). Breast cancer: An artistic view. *The Lancet, 8*, 583–585.
van Prooijen, J.-W., & Douglas, K. M. (2017). Conspiracy theories as part of history: The role of societal crisis situations. *Memory Studies, 10*(3), 323–333.

von Engelhardt, D. (2021). Cancer in literature: Between phenomenology and symbolism. In A. W. Bauer, R.-D. Hofheinz, & J. S. Utikal (Eds.), *Ethical challenges in cancer diagnosis and treatment* (pp. 275–290). Springer.

Wadler, J. (1992). *My breast.* Pocket Books.

Wagoner, B. (2015). Collective remembering as a process of social representation. In G. Sammut, E. Andreouli, G. Gaskell, & J. Valsiner (Eds.), *The Cambridge handbook of social representations* (pp. 143–162). Cambridge University Press.

WHO. (2025). *WHO COVID-19 dashboard. COVID-19 deaths|WHO COVID-19 dashboard.*

Winskell, K. (2021). Social representations theory and young Africans' creative narratives about HIV/AIDS, 1997–2014. *Journal for the Theory of Social Behaviour, 51*(1), 164–182.

Winskell, K., Brown, P. J., Patterson, A. E., & Mbakwem, B. L. (2013). Making sense of HIV/AIDS in Southeast Nigeria: Fictional narratives, cultural meanings and methodologies in medical anthropology. *Medical Anthropology Quarterly, 27*(2), 193–214.

Winskell, K., & Enger, D. (2014). Storytelling for social change: Reflections on narrative and narration in global health communication. In K. G. Wilkins, T. Tufte, & R. Obregon (Eds.), *Handbook of developmental communication and social change* (pp. 189–206). Wiley-Blackwell.

Winskell, K., Singleton, R., Sibben, G., Tiendrebeogo, G., Obong'o, C., Dia, F. L., & et al. (2020). Social representations of the prevention of heterosexual transmission of HIV among young Africans from five countries, 1997–2014. *PLoS One, 15* (3), e02278878.

CHAPTER 7

Health and Illness Among Older People

The Western world is experiencing increasing longevity in its population. People are living longer, and there are more older people. It is estimated that within the next 25 years, the number of people aged 60 and more will have doubled. This has led to sustained public discussion about the social and health implications of the changing demographics of our societies. A series of studies have explored social representations of health and illness among older people. This chapter contrasts the more work-oriented older residents of Aberdeen in the north-east of Scotland with the more lifestyle-oriented baby-boomers of Canada. It concludes by considering a study of the social representations of older people held by health professionals in Germany. It also explores the socio-historic location of the different research studies.

7.1 Growing Older

The Western world is experiencing increasing longevity in its population. This has involved a transition from the acceptance of chronology as the primary indicator of ageing to greater attention to social and psychological processes. There is a questioning of the assumption that the loss of function is the inevitable consequence of ageing and consideration of the factors that enhance or hinder the quality of life for older people (Walker, 2014).

M. Murray, *Social Representations, Health and Illness*,
https://doi.org/10.1007/978-3-031-98494-5_7

This raises the question as to the nature of ageing. From a biological perspective, it can be considered as damage to cells and tissues; from a physiological perspective, it can be more about changes in organ functions, while to the clinician, it can be concerned with increasing frailty and the development of various diseases (Cox et al., 2014). However, from a psychological perspective, ageing can be concerned with the varying experiences as you grow older, while from a social perspective, it is more concerned with the broader social and cultural processes. From a social psychological perspective, the focus is on the changing character of everyday social interaction and on the social representations of ageing.

Images of the ageing person have figured in art and literature since ancient times. Artistic portrayals of old people appear in portraits, historical accounts, allegories and many other genres. In particular, 'the aged male body is the distinguishing mark of patriarchs, prophets, hermits, or scholars in Biblical scenes, or it might denote philosophers of antiquity' (Kampmann, 2015, p. 280). One particular feature of artistic representation of ageing is its historical and gender specificity. While men have historically been portrayed in terms of power, with women in terms of subservience, this has changed over time. Since at least the sixteenth century, women have been portrayed in terms of their bodies, sexuality and motherhood. Von Hülsen-Esch (2022) has commented on the misogynistic images of older women since the Middle Ages.

In the modern era, images of older people circulate in the mass media, including advertising, film, television and the internet. These images both reflect contemporary views of ageing and contribute to the content of social representations. However, while contemporary images are important, the more classical images of earlier eras continue to resonate.

The physical portrayal of older people in public images can range from 'ageing gracefully' to 'mutton dressed as lamb' (Fairhurst, 1998). This is particularly the case with portrayals of women. Images can promote certain views of older people, but they can also subvert certain traditional images. For example, older people can be portrayed as engaging in activities traditionally associated with younger people. It all depends on the production and reception context (Kaufman, 1994). What was the intention of the producer, and what was the expectation of the audience?

Representations of older people in the media and the arts continue to change. A study in the 1990s found that older adults, especially women, were rarely portrayed in the media, often rendering them invisible. When they were portrayed, they were presented as ugly, senile, ill and less friendly, as well as less sexually active (Vernon et al., 1991). A more recent analysis of popular television shows revealed a much-changed representation. Old age was presented as a time of transition when new opportunities could be found. Older characters were more often portrayed as wise but also as funny or striving to gain the wisdom that they lacked (Waltz & Gran, 2017). Women are also a particular target of the pharmaceutical industry, with widespread promotion of cosmetic products supposedly designed to delay the aging process (Warren, 2018).

Literature is also filled with conflicting images of ageing. Traditionally, literature represented the old person in negative terms and the process of ageing as one of a lack of social engagement and withdrawal. However, contemporary literature often challenges such images. The classic image of decline in both physical and mental capacity is epitomized in the description written 400 years ago by Shakespeare of the sixth age, when the old (male) person moves into 'the lean and slippered pantaloon,/ With spectacles on nose and pouch on side;/ His youthful hose, well saved, a world too wide/ For his shrunk shank, and his big manly voice,/ Turning again towards childish treble, pipes/ And whistles in his sound'. This is before the last scene of all, which he describes as 'second childishness and mere oblivion,/ Sans teeth, sans eyes, sans taste, sans everything'. This image is increasingly challenged.

Older people play much more important and prominent roles in contemporary literature. This might be a reflection of the aging readership demanding such roles or publishers finding a growing market among the expanding ageing demographic. Another feature is the evidence that authors are increasingly continuing to write into old age, and their novels reflect that experience (Hepworth, 2000).

This is indeed the case with academics. Erikson (1997) noted in her preface to *The Life Cycle Completed* the pleasures and opportunities of a ninth stage of human development in late old age, about which her husband (Erik Erikson) had not written. While she accepted the physical decline of her body, she reckoned that old age offers a more positive trajectory for the elderly, guided by hope and faith. A study by Graham Crow of retired academics found that 'continuing scholars' is a frequent route taken by many academics after retirement through continued involvement in different scholarly activities (Crow, 2021). Their opportunity to pursue these activities depended upon the reception and support provided. The changing societal expectations were evident in studies of social representations of ageing.

7.2 Growing Older in 1970s Scotland

The 1970s was a period of sustained change in northern Scotland. Aberdeen, the major city in the region, had traditionally been dependent on the fishing industry, shipbuilding, and the textile trade. It was a strongly Presbyterian society accustomed to austerity, hard work and a conservative lifestyle, as well as a strong commitment to military service, especially among men. Then, in the 1970s, oil was discovered in the North Sea, and Aberdeen became the new oil capital of Britain, with increasing wealth and a more cosmopolitan lifestyle. However, older people still held on to their traditional values.

The trilogy, *A Scots Quair*, by Lewis Grassic Gibbon (2006), is regarded as a classic sequence of novels describing changes in twentieth-century Scotland. It consists of three novels—*Sunset Song*, *Cloud Howe* and *Grey Granite*—and graphically details the changing circumstances of north-east Scotland as the characters move from a rural to an urban life. Gibbon describes the importance of work in the lives of the characters, the impact of World War, and the poverty experienced by many. He also details the central role of religion and politics in his characters' lives. In *Grey Granite,* one of the characters reflected on the endemic poverty: 'She had nothing at all, she had never had anything, nothing in the world she'd believed in but change ... Nothing endured'.

The sense of ongoing tenacity in the face of hardship and change was reflected in the accounts of older Aberdonians collected by Rory Williams. In 1978–1980, Williams, a sociologist, conducted a detailed study of understandings of health, illness and ageing among older residents of Aberdeen (Williams, 1983). This intensive study involved detailed biographical interviews with a sample of 70 older people, supplemented with a larger survey study of over 600 participants. In analysing the interview transcripts, Williams compared his findings with those of Herzlich (1973).

He organized the older people's understandings of health into three categories: *health as the absence of disease,* which was similar to Herzlich's 'health as not illness' (which Williams described as the mechanical level); *health as a continuum of strength,* which was similar to Herzlich's 'health as reserve' (the personal level) and *health as being fit* or *able for it,* which was similar to Herzlich's 'health as equilibrium' (or the social level). However, there were certain differences, especially in the last category. In Aberdeen the old people emphasized the importance of being fit and able to fulfil everyday obligations, whereas in France it was about maintaining an equilibrium with one's way of life. While in Scotland this fitness was premised on the absence of sickness, in France it was based upon a reserve of health and strength. It was suggested that the more frequent use of the term 'equilibrium' in Herzlich's study echoed a more middle-class way of coping with life in France or reflected the middle-class composition of her sample.

There was also a difference in the second category, which in the Scottish sample was a continuum from strength to weakness. This, in some ways, is an intermediate state—neither healthy nor ill—but in Scotland, weakness did not justify people saying that they were unfit for their normal obligations. Conversely, in Herzlich's study, there was frequent reference to fatigue and vulnerability, which could upset the equilibrium. Thus, while in Scotland, feeling unwell did not mean you could not work, in France, it led to a reduction in normal activity.

Williams (1990) pursued these ideas further in his analysis of the participants' understanding of illness, ageing and death. He emphasized the strong Presbyterian heritage of his study participants. Their understandings of illness were organized into five categories: (a) illness as controlled by normal living, (b) illness as a continuous struggle, (c) illness as an alternative way of life, (d) illness as a loss to be endured and (e) illness as a release from effort. Again, he compared these categories with Herzlich's threefold classification. Combining (a) continued normal living and (d) illness to be endured was similar to *illness as a destroyer*. This combination of continued performance of normal responsibilities with a certain sense of helplessness was labelled *illness as exile*. The second pattern, which combined (a) continued normal living with (b) continuous struggle, was similar to *illness as occupation* and was labelled *illness as a test of achievement*. A difference with the French study was that the Aberdonians had an optimistic view of the health-giving properties of normal living. These two patterns contrasted resignation with resistance. The third pattern, which combined (d) illness to be endured and (e) illness as release, was similar to *illness as liberator* and was labelled *illness as disengagement*. This view was unusual among the Aberdonians and was largely understood in terms of rest and release rather than a new opportunity. Instead, it was felt that continuing with normal activities was the preferred approach to illness.

Underlying these understandings of illness, which the Aberdonians combined in different ways, were two broad concepts of health—the moral and the mechanical. The moral approach emphasized that the normal way of life was health-giving, and people are responsible for its maintenance.

The mechanical approach accepted that certain restrictions were imposed by the body. There was a social pressure to conform and to continue with normal life. This moral approach to health reflected the participants' approach to work and life. As Williams (1990) summarized their feelings on being excluded from social and work life, they were 'lost', no longer themselves, 'socially dead', 'finished'. Their strong work ethic combined with a moral value of helping others, which brought with it a reward of health and reflected the older participants' Presbyterian heritage.

In their discussion of ageing, the older people emphasized the importance of their generation's heritage of wartime deprivation and economic austerity. This had contributed to their valuing 'hard work, courage, effort and activity, an ability to be satisfied with little, and the thrift to make a little go a long way'. Their views on ageing were grouped into three categories: retirement, illness and the death of contemporaries. While ageing was sometimes grounds for retirement, it could also be a consequence of retirement.

Ageing was initially classified into five categories: (a) early old age as liberation, (b) early old age as a setback, (c) early old age as the repairing of defences, (d) late old age as resistible and (e) late old age as a surrender. These five categories were combined into three categories: ageing as a *resurgence*, as *a siege* and as *delayed capitulation*. Resurgence involved liberation from previous restrictions, the repairing of defences and resisting late old age. Siege involved seeing early old age as a setback but also as an opportunity for repairing defences and resisting late old age. The most common pattern was delayed capitulation, which viewed early old age as a setback and as an opportunity for repairing defences but late old age as a surrender. Illness was seen as almost an inevitable consequence of entry into this final stage.

Thus, early old age was seen as both a time of opportunity and a time of resistance. The more middle-class participants especially emphasized the opportunities. Late old age was seen as a stage to be pitied, involving living beyond the normal time to die. In some ways, late old age was a discredited identity that required segregation. It was a stage to be avoided, if possible—for example, by not participating in activities designed for older people. There were two broad perspectives: the more pessimistic viewed ageing as inevitable, whereas the more optimistic emphasized the moral tradition of work and effort. Williams concluded that it reflected Scottish Calvinism, with its emphasis on action to overcome evil.

For these older people, health was anchored in their ability to work. These older Aberdonians placed great value on work, and they inherited a consciousness from war and economic depression, which gave rise to a particular view of work distinct from that of young people. As Williams (1990) noted, 'The seriousness thus accorded to work, to take days off even for illness, sometimes even to do no part-time work after retirement, was inherently a dubious decision' (p. 226). For many women of this generation, housekeeping was their work, and they regarded it seriously. Hard work had a moral value.

This was coupled with the strong Calvinist approach within Scottish Presbyterianism, which placed a strong value on hard work. Religion also gave a sense of identity, which supported a communitarian ethic of helping those in need. Among those older people who adopted a strong ethical view of life, 'control of health was not just by personal powers of character, but by personal rules of good living; not drinking, not smoking, being actively involved in helping people' (Williams, 1990, p. 292). Religion could also provide a meaning to suffering, as you could gain from it. Clean living was next to godliness and could not only preserve health but also delay ageing.

7.3 Growing Older in Canada in the 2000s

Like many Western societies, Canadian society is currently going through a major demographic change as a result of the aging of the so-called baby-boomers—those individuals who were born in the period immediately following the Second World War. In most Western societies, there was a steady increase in births in the aftermath of that war. In the 20-year period after the Second World War, there was a bulge in the population of North America and other countries due to the increased birth rate. In Canada, the birth rate rose from 24.3 per 1000 in 1945 to 26.8 in 1960 and then fell to 17.5 in 1970 (Foot, 1999). At that time, there was sustained political debate about the implications of the baby-boom population reaching retirement.

These so-called baby-boomers began to come of adult age in the late 1960s, a period of relative affluence after war-time restrictions. It was also the period of liberalization of social policies and expansion of the welfare system. This was the period when the Canadian national identity was clearly defined with the adoption of the Maple Leaf flag, the implementation of official bilingualism and multiculturalism, comprehensive healthcare and extensive higher education. In literature, writers such as Robertson Davies, Mordechai Richler and then Margaret Atwood signalled the arrival of the nation on the international cultural scene. The introduction of Canadian content regulations on television and radio around this time was designed to preserve and promote Canadian cultural identity. In popular music, Canadian singers became prominent internationally. These included Leonard Cohen, Joni Mitchel and Neil Young, one of whose famous songs titled *Old Man (Look at My Life)* from his 1972 album *Harvest* reflected on the ageing process. The popular band Steppenwolf included two Canadian members. It became world-famous with their song *Born to Be Wild* (1968), which featured in the popular film *Easy Rider* (1969). The lyrics of the song ('We were born, born to be wild/We can climb so high/I never want to die') conveyed the quest for immortality that fascinated this generation.

As they entered their 50s, this ageing population began to turn to the health service for support as their health and that of their parents started to falter. In view of their increased life expectancy, there was growing political debate about the implications for the cost of health and social care.

The late 1900s was a period in Canada when the government introduced a range of measures designed to promote health and treat illness. In 1974, the government released a report entitled *A New Perspective on the Health of Canadians* (Lalonde, 1974). This document, known as the Lalonde Report after Marc Lalonde, the Minister of Health, became foundational for the development of the concept of health promotion. It identified four elements of what was defined as the 'health field': human biology, environment, lifestyle and healthcare. Improvements in health required action on the environment, healthcare and lifestyle. The publication of this report was followed by a wide range of government and federal initiatives designed to promote health, especially through lifestyle and behaviour change initiatives.

This was followed by the convening of an International Conference in Ottawa in 1984 by the World Health Organization, which issued the *Ottawa Charter for Health Promotion* (WHO, 1986). This charter set out the principles for actions designed to improve the health of populations through health promotion. This action had five strands: building healthy public policy; creating supportive environments; strengthening community action; developing personal skills and re-orienting healthcare services towards the prevention of illness and the promotion of health (Potvin & Jones, 2011). In the same year, the 'Canada Health Act' reaffirmed a publicly funded healthcare system that provided a comprehensive range of health services for all citizens. This was an extremely popular measure, reflected in the fact that it was passed unopposed in the national parliament (Tiedemann, 2019).

However, in the 1990s, at a time of growing austerity internationally, more conservative elements in the parliament began to express concern about the cost of the health system. This was followed in 2001 by the establishment of a Royal Commission on the Future of Health Care in Canada. This commission was named the Romanow Commission after its chair, Roy Romanow, a former Premier of the province of Saskatchewan. The Commission produced its final report, titled *Building on Values: The Future of Health Care in Canada*, in 2002 (Romanow, 2002). This report confirmed the central role of a publicly funded healthcare system with various steps to improve efficiency and address inequalities in access (Browne, 2004). It was around this time that a study of social representations of health and illness among baby-boomers in Canada was launched.

The *Norms and Narratives Study* (Murray et al., 1999) was a large study of the beliefs about health, illness, ageing and healthcare held by baby-boomers in Canada. In the full study, over 500 men and women from a range of different social and ethnic backgrounds, drawn from urban and rural regions across Canada, participated in individual or group discussions about health, illness, ageing and healthcare. Participants were recruited initially through community agencies and subsequently through a marketing agency to reflect a cross-section of middle-aged men and women from different social backgrounds. Those group participants recruited by the marketing agency received a small fee for their participation. The group discussions were preferred as the prime method of data collection as they allowed the participants much greater control over setting the agenda, besides revealing more clearly the extent to which the views expressed were shared by peers (cf. Caillaud et al., 2022). These group discussions were supplemented with individual interviews that provided an opportunity for participants to expand upon particular personal experiences.

The discussions followed a series of broad themes and encouraged the participants to reflect on their experiences of health, illness, ageing and healthcare. Following the episodic interview format (Flick, 1992), the participants were encouraged to consider their own personal experiences of health, illness and healthcare. The participants were eager to describe their experiences and express their viewpoints, thus requiring the facilitators to play only a minor role.

All the discussions were tape-recorded, transcribed and entered onto a database where they were broadly coded. Subsequently, the authors read and re-read sections of the discussions to clarify how particular concepts were expressed. These concepts were sometimes not apparent in single quotes but in an exchange between members of a discussion group, illustrating how ideas are developed and shared in the interaction. They were also filled with examples from the participants' lives.

This study was conducted across the whole of Canada, but the discussion here is largely limited to the part conducted in the Eastern provinces of Newfoundland, New Brunswick, Prince Edward Island and Nova Scotia (Murray et al., 2003). A total of 154 participants, aged 45–55 years, were recruited for the study in that region. Most were involved in one of 20 discussion groups, plus 28 who participated in individual interviews. The participants reflected a cross-section of men ($n = 62$) and women ($n = 92$) from different socio-economic backgrounds.

7.3.1 Health, Illness and Healthcare

Representations of health: These were initially classified into six dimensions: *lifestyle, attitude, social engagement, reserve, functionality* and *vacuum*. The primary definition was in terms of a *healthy lifestyle*. This was something at which you had to continuously work. The more middle-class participants emphasized this dimension. For example, one woman said:

> I don't think being healthy is something you ever arrive at. I think it's something you're always … you're working at, always striving to improve but you're slipping a bit and you're trying to regain ground and things happen and you're recovering from that and so on. So it really is … like it's a lifelong process working at trying to stay healthy; and sometimes you're more healthier than others and sometimes, you know, you slip back and … regain ground … You can't … your body is always changing and you're always … you know. It's not constant. So you have to educate yourself about the changes that your body is going through in order for you to stay healthy.

Some of the more middle-class men felt that younger people were healthier because they had internalized this healthy lifestyle message, whereas in their own generation, it had been acceptable to behave in an unhealthy manner. They also emphasized the role of parents. As one middle-class man said:

> I mean, you know, I think they're going to be a lot healthier from now in the next 25 years – the small kids – because they got good parents. Good parents are going to tell them, you shouldn't drink. You shouldn't smoke. You shouldn't do drugs. You shouldn't do this because we know now. *We* didn't know before because there was no …

Working-class participants agreed on the importance of lifestyle but also felt that it was difficult to adopt healthy lifestyle practices. As one working man said: 'The attitude also—I'll start … I'll start tomorrow. Tomorrow comes, aw, next week maybe'.

Related to lifestyle was *health as attitude*. This was a person's attitude or general orientation to life—how a person dealt with various aspects of daily life. Thus, you could have some health problems, but you could still be healthy because of having a positive attitude. As one woman said:

> I could be crippled and be very healthy. I could have my arm removed and be very healthy. I could sit here today and be quite sick because my quality of life is gone. I'm feeling miserable. I'm lonely. I'm scared. To me health is far broader than I've got a stomach ache or a cold. It's the way my life appears to me and I think, as a I say, I could be in a wheelchair and be an extremely healthy person but I could also be sitting here tonight and if I'm depressed and I'm lonely and I'm scared …

The importance of attitude was particularly pronounced among the middle-class participants.

Then there was *health as social engagement*. It was felt that having strong family and community relationships protected one from illness. Those individuals who had strong social and family ties were considered healthy. As one man said: 'If someone has a sense of wellbeing, whether it's involved in family relationships or connections to the community, that really is the key'.

The fourth theme was *health as a reserve*. This was concerned with the extent to which the person had a healthy constitution. Thus, as one man said: 'I sometimes think that it depends on the genes in a lot of families and there somethings that seem to be prevalent in families, like heart attacks ...' An important component of this reserve was being born with a healthy constitution, although this could be compromised by a problematic upbringing. One woman described this: 'Some people have just horrendous life situations to deal with—through no fault of their own, too'. This upbringing could impact later health.

The fifth theme was *health as functionality* or the ability to continue working despite some health problems. For example, one man said: 'As long as I can go to work and not feel too bad and have a good time and not be hospitalised for anything ...' But the ability to continue working and functioning in everyday life depended on having a sense of purpose. As one man said: 'I think that's ... to me, that's three-quarters of being healthy is to have a purpose, have something that takes your mind off yourself for one thing and makes you think of ... somebody else and what you got to do'.

The sixth dimension was simply the absence of illness or health in a *vacuum*. Taken together, these themes represent a very modernist conception of health as something that could be achieved through good living, having friends and a sense of purpose.

These six dimensions could be compared with Herzlich's three categories. Health in a vacuum was similar to Herzlich's, as was health as reserve. Health as social engagement and functionality was similar to Herzlich's equilibrium. The two remaining categories, lifestyle and attitude, are additional categories and reflect the importance of lifestyle and personal responsibility for health, which had been emphasized in government health promotion programmes in Canada.

Representations of illness: There were two primary dimensions of illness: *destruction* and *struggle*. The *destruction* dimension emphasized the negative impact of illness on your life. An example of the destructive impact on life was given by a male professional in an individual interview:

> Now I have got a thing called eye trouble that came on about a year and half ago. That is the patch here; it is just to prevent me from seeing double because my eyes were playing tricks. And that is an aspect of it. So it kind of dealt me a pretty hard blow a year and a half ago. I went through probably two or three months getting a grip on it. So there was anxiety and things of that nature, and trying to deal with the physical symptoms as well. So I spent a kind of miserable few months full of self-pity, fear, doubt. It is probably

> a good example of how one's attitude can change from being in charge to one of I don't know what is going to happen and I think I could be totally dependent on others and helpless and that sort of thing.

This account was labelled 'destruction' because the participant described going from 'being in charge' to being 'totally dependent'. However, the participant could escape this destruction by 'getting a grip on it'. This opportunity to escape overlaps with the second dimension.

The *struggle* dimension was concerned with working to overcome the limitations imposed by having an illness. For example, one middle-class woman recounted the experience of a colleague who had developed breast cancer.

> She, I think, had both breasts removed and then a recurrence of cancer in the last two years of her life and it metastasized. What I saw with her was ... there was anger and an edge, you know, which may have been part of her personality but a sense of she'd been burdened with things that she wouldn't have chosen and that, in many ways, her life was full of [...]; and yet, at the same time, she was willing to do whatever to give her some time because she had young ... she had children [...] you need that kind of spunk, and so I think energy can come from that.

The struggle was related to the fact that this woman had children, and as was mentioned in the previous chapter, responsibility for children is of prime importance for married women.

There was no reference to illness as a *liberator*. In all of the discussions, the participants stressed the negative aspects of illness. It was something that threatened their quality of life, and the aim was to overcome it. Unlike Herzlich's study, none of the participants in this study reported serious health problems and thus did not have the opportunity to reflect on the liberation dimension of illness, although this was apparent in discussions of ageing.

Causes of illness: There were four primary causes of illness: *lifestyle, self-care, nature* and *modern life*. *Lifestyle* included a range of behaviours considered a threat to health, e.g., 'My aunt ... smoked and drank—two big no-nos. She killed herself the same way my father-in-law did'. The person was responsible for these behaviours as he/she was for *self-care*, e.g., 'Some people may have brought it on themselves through, you know, not being careful'. Conversely, there was the view that illness was part of

nature, of being human. One man said: 'People do get sick. No matter how much healthy food you eat, you still get sick. It's just the animal nature'. Finally, some participants referred to the stress of ***modern life***, e.g., 'In this world today, there is a lot of stress'.

Again, there was the tension between the individual and society. The individual was generally healthy, but the stresses and strains of modern life threatened this health. In addition, there was the need to maintain good health by adopting a healthy lifestyle and looking after yourself. These activities could prevent illness. There was an increasing awareness of the importance of taking responsibility for your health. As one man said:

> And there was a lot of advertising about promoting and encouraging people to get out and be more physically active and amount of exercise and to get involved in things. To be careful about your diet, don't drink too much, don't smoke. All these types of messages that are out there now, that weren't out there say 25 years ago. Everybody who doesn't practice this stuff can't state that they are not doing the proper thing because they are ignorant of what the proper thing is. There is real choices that you shouldn't ignore all these messages about your health.

Connecting health and illness: The representations of health and illness are complementary. This is illustrated in Table 7.1. Being healthy meant having a good lifestyle, while illness was caused by a poor lifestyle. This was the activity definition of health and illness. Similarly, health was a positive attitude, and illness was poor self-care. Health as reserve emphasized a person's constitution, while illness was something intrinsically wrong with the person. All three of these dimensions were internal or

Table 7.1 Definitions of health and illness

Health	*Illness cause*	*Illness character*	*Illness prevention*
Lifestyle	Lifestyle	Destruction	Healthy lifestyle
Attitude	Self-care	Struggle	Self-care
Reserve	Nature		
Social engagement	Modern life		
Functionality			
Vacuum			

Source Murray and Rodgers (2002).

endogenous, while modern life was external and similar to Herzlich's way of life.

Together, this understanding of health was framed in terms of a healthy lifestyle, which was seen as everyone's responsibility. These accounts were presented in a narrative form, detailing personal examples of people who neglected adopting a healthy lifestyle. As in Herzlich's study, there was a tension between lifestyle and modern society. While the government promoted a healthy lifestyle, many of the participants felt that the modern way of life curtailed their ability to adopt it. An important aspect was their perceived responsibility as Canadian citizens. Good citizens would follow government guidance on health promotion. Thus, the social representation of health as a healthy lifestyle implied a social identity of a good Canadian citizen; it was right and proper to adopt a healthy lifestyle.

Healthcare: This issue of identity was also apparent in their representations of healthcare (Murray & Rodgers, 2002). The dominant view among the participants was that a socialized, publicly funded healthcare system, as it existed in Canada, was the best. As one man said:

> We want universal medical care—to go back is uncivilized. Well, basically, it raises your ... what you think a civilized nation should be when you have that and you don't want to go back after that ... also, because you think that everybody deserves it.

The character of Canadian healthcare was something of which they were very proud. It was a system based on equal access and free at the point of use. This system was described as civilized and was what differentiated Canada from the United States. This point was repeatedly emphasized in the group discussions. As one man said: 'It wasn't put in for the rich people. It was put in for the poor people to have the same amount'. Another added: 'I care about my fellow Canadians'.

As baby-boomers, they were very proud of the healthcare system, which they had supported since its creation and were now increasingly using. For them, it was a mark of a civilized society based upon fairness and social justice. This was the Canada which they had helped to shape in their lifetimes. The healthcare system was a characteristic of Canada that distinguished it from the United States, which was seen as uncivilized. Canada was a society based upon support for each other. However, the participants foresaw certain problems in financing the system as they aged and made increasing use of it. As one man said:

> I think we got the greatest system in the whole world what I can see. But now is how, and I see why we're here tonight trying to maybe foresee a problem coming and it would be sad to see it go like everybody's opinion is and my opinion is the same because we're going to be baby boomers who are going to get sick, I imagine. We're going to need pills. We're after 50.

7.3.2 *Old or Older*

Growing old was described in terms of a tension between the ageing person and society. Age was reflected in terms of: (a) a *deterioration* in physical appearance and ability, (b) a *journey* in managing ageing, (c) a new *opportunity* and (d) a growing awareness of *death*. These four categories are similar to Herzlich's threefold classification of illness *as destruction, occupation* and *liberation*, with the added category of *death*. The character of growing older was also dependent on the attitude of society. These categories are detailed in Table 7.2.

Deterioration was the decline of physical capacity, which was apparent in physical appearance and limitations across four components. The second main category was described as the *journey* of ageing. This was concerned with how people managed the process of ageing. This was similar to the struggle description of illness but less acute because it was not a short-term event but a long-term process. For some of the boomers, an awareness of ageing provided an *opportunity* to reassess life's priorities. This was most apparent among the middle-class participants who had taken early retirement. The fourth category was concerned with increasing *awareness of death*, which was the ultimate destruction of life. It was something that the baby-boomers began to think about. Growing old meant a tension with *societal expectations* and norms. It was felt that older people were often excluded from opportunities, made to feel a burden on society and generally treated with disrespect in everyday social interaction.

Table 7.2 Social representations of ageing

Deterioration	Physical appearance, aches and pains, physical limitations, illness
Journey	Denial, attitude, lifestyle, finances, independence
Opportunity	Achievement, no worries, new activities
Death	Inevitability, death of peers, attitude toward death
Society	Excluded, burden, labelled

Source Murray and Rodgers (2002)

The baby-boomers were very keen to emphasize that they were not old, but they accepted that they were growing older. When they were younger, being 50 years old was considered old, but now they did not want to consider 80 years old to be old. They were frustrated by the various attempts to label people aged over 50 as being old.

7.3.3 Lifestyle and Identity

A common theme in these social representations of health, illness and ageing among the baby-boomers in Canada was lifestyle and social engagement. Health was associated with an active lifestyle and social engagement, while illness was linked to a poor lifestyle and neglecting self-care, resulting in social exclusion. Health was anchored in a healthy lifestyle and social activity. For ageing, similar concepts were used, but there was a growing awareness of the inevitability of physical changes in the body as a result of ageing. The physical appearance of older individuals deteriorated, and they became less physically active. Ageing was anchored in a decline in physical activity and social engagement, although this could be contested by maintaining an active lifestyle and practicing self-care.

A similar classification of illness and ageing was apparent. There was physical, personal and social deterioration as the old person was less able to participate in various activities. However, this was not inevitable; it depended upon the attitude of the older person and the opportunities provided by society. An important aspect was the issue of identity as a Canadian citizen and as an older person. These were the baby-boomers who had lived through the period of rising prosperity in Canada, the development of universal healthcare, and the promotion of healthy lifestyles. These developments were part of the Canadian identity, of which they were proud.

From a discursive perspective, the study participants were engaged in presenting an image of the good Canadian. The hegemonic social representation of health emphasized taking care of yourself and promoting health. The participants felt that they were good Canadians and through their healthy lifestyle portraying that identity.

7.4 Older People in Germany in the 2000s

As in the rest of the Western world, Germany has experienced sustained increases in life expectancy over the past 50 years and is expected to continue increasing at a rate of 1.5 years per decade. Coupled with this is the increasing proportion of the population over 60 years, and it is expected that by 2030 the proportion of the population classified as elderly will have reached 30–40%. The rapid increase in the number of older people has led to discussions regarding the implications for government services. As they age, older people have more contact with healthcare and various health professionals. It was estimated that while older people currently represent 25% of general practitioners' patients, they account for 40% of treatment contacts (Flick et al., 2002).

Germany has a comprehensive healthcare service dating back to the introduction of the Health Insurance Bill by Otto von Bismarck, the first Chancellor of Germany, in 1883. This service was based on the principles of solidarity (access for all), subsidiarity (minimal political influence) and corporatism (relationship between government and health professions). The majority of services are funded through statutory and private health insurance.

After the horrors of the Second World War, Germany was divided into a capitalist free-market West and a communist East. However, they were re-united in 1991, and the country is now a major economic power in the world. The denazification of the country was accompanied by the promotion of American consumer culture while maintaining elements of German classical culture. It was also a culture that embraced technology.

It was in this context of political change and increasing debate about healthcare that Uwe Flick and his colleagues conducted a study of health professionals' social representations of the health of older people in Germany (Flick et al., 2003). In this study, a sample of general practitioners and home-care nurses from Berlin and Hamburg (former West Germany) participated in individual episodic interviews about health in old age. Thematic analysis of these interviews identified three broad categories: *situation of living*, *management of disease and complaints* and character of any *disease and complaints*. Each of these categories had several sub-categories. These are summarized in Table 7.3.

The major finding was that health professionals agreed that health was more than the absence of physical symptoms and could be present even when someone had a chronic disease. It all depended on the living

Table 7.3 Professional concepts of health in old age

Situation of living	Independence, self-determination, autonomy, mobility, quality of life, social integration, receipt of support, mental activity, vitality
Management of disease	Arrange (adjust to) symptoms and restrictions, meaningfulness despite restrictions, subjective vs. objective health, satisfaction in spite of complaints
Disease and complaints	Prevention, living with decline, capacity, medical problems, absence of chronic disease, absence of complaints and pain

Source Flick et al. (2003)

arrangements of the individual concerned. There were certain similarities with the organization of social representations of health suggested by Herzlich (1973). The first category of the *situation of living* was similar to Herzlich's *equilibrium,* with its emphasis on activity and social relations. The second main category was the *management of disease*, which was similar to Herzlich's *reserve of health*, including *resistance to attacks* as a feature. Thus, health was conceived as a sort of reservoir that could manage the onset of chronic disease or pain. The third category included details of *disease and complaints* that the person could live with, which could be compared with Herzlich's category of *health in a vacuum*. There was little reference to *health as a lifestyle,* which may have been due to the fact that these health professionals did not consider this important among older people.

Overall, these German health professionals had moved beyond the classic biomedical definition of health and had developed a social representation of health for older people that was attuned to ideas promoted by the World Health Organization. The focus was less on the absence of disease and more on the extent of social activity among older people, their ability to adjust to restrictions, and maintain a degree of autonomy and self-determination. It was also similar to Herzlich's work, with its emphasis on the importance of activity but also on the management of any complaints, perhaps reflecting the health professionals' concerns about excessive use of healthcare. Flick et al. noted at the onset that older people have regular contact with their family doctors and that traditional lifestyle strategies are less relevant for them. The alternative, more social approach, is to promote greater social engagement among older people.

7.5 Anchoring Health in Work

While the social representations of health, illness and ageing among the Aberdonians were informed by a strong Presbyterian work ethic, among the Canadian baby-boomers, it was informed more by a social gospel. Among the Aberdonians, there was a commitment to fulfilling social obligations through work and community support. Williams (1990) described this as a moral approach to health. The older people were committed to playing a role in society. As they aged, they felt no longer able to do this. They struggled to maintain active engagement but eventually succumbed due to physical limitations.

This is complemented by the German health professionals' managerial approach to health and illness (Flick et al., 2002). It was their job to keep people engaged in society. This was part of the broader German ethic of the centrality of work in life and the need to carefully manage resources. While this work ethic is often traced back to the rise of Protestantism in the sixteenth century, its secularized version is more commonplace today. The emphasis was on work as a virtue and leisure as a moral threat, or as Max Weber (1864–1920) said in *The Protestant Ethic and the Spirit of Capitalism* (1904–5): 'Loss of time through sociability, idle talk, luxury, even more sleep than is necessary for health, six to at most eight hours, is worthy of absolute condemnation' (in Just, 2014). Commitment to work had to be applied to all aspects of daily life.

This commitment to work was evident in other prominent German philosophers, including Hegel and Marx (Just, 2014). Hegel considered work the foundation of human culture. However, Marx criticized what he considered the idealized approach of Hegel, with his focus on spiritual work. Instead, he argued for the centrality of material work. While this material work was central to Marx's conception of humanity, it was jeopardized in capitalist society, where the ruling class owned the means of production such that the working person felt alienated from their labour. Still, there remained the push for humanity to regain the real value of work through various endeavours.

The ideas of John Calvin (1509–1564) were particularly influential in the development of the Protestant Reformation in the sixteenth century. Calvin not only lauded the value of work but also emphasized the need for self-denial and caring for one's neighbour. As he said: 'When scripture tells us to put aside selfish interests, it not only removes undue desire for wealth, power or popularity from our minds, but wipes out all ambition for worldly glory' (Calvin, in Eaton, 2013, p. 3). Calvin's austere ideas were further developed in Scotland by John Knox (1514–1572). These ideas were also supported by the growth of Freemasonry in Scotland, with its themes of brotherhood, equality and hard work (Smith, 2009).

The Protestant Reformation in Scotland was followed in the eighteenth century by the Scottish Enlightenment, which promoted virtue and wisdom. This ideology emphasized the idea that people are not entitled to happiness but must attain it through hard work and merit. This melding of religious ideas with economic and intellectual progress continues to infuse Scottish society (Smith, 2009). For the older Aberdonians, ageing held up the prospect of new forms of work, which often involved participation in voluntary organizations. It was through these new forms of work that they could maintain health and wellbeing. They were Scottish, and part of this identity was a commitment to work. Illness was not a liberator but more a rest from these work obligations, to which one would eventually return. Old age, however, held out the prospect of physical deterioration and restricted ability. Health was anchored in the ability to work, which was central to their identity.

Among the Canadian baby-boomers, health was more about fulfilling a broad social obligation to maintain a healthy lifestyle, which in some way was the new religion. They were proud of their Canadian identity and felt they had a role to play in supporting the benefits of the society that they had helped to build. The social gospel of helping and supporting those in need was an intrinsic part of their Canadian identity, as was maintaining their health.

Religion was not mentioned by the boomers, although Christian religions have been prominent in Canadian history. A 2019 survey found that two-thirds of Canadians reported having a religious affiliation, and a large proportion reported that their religious beliefs were important in their lives. Although there has been an overall decline in formal religious affiliation among boomers, it remains high (Cornelissen, 2021). The dominant religion in Canada has been Christianity, infused with a social concern for others. This religion was more in terms of humanism rather than spirituality. It was the Christian socialism of the baby-boomers' generation which had promoted the development of the Canadian healthcare system. This system was formally initiated in the prairie province of Saskatchewan by the social democrat politician Tommy Douglas, who was voted the *Greatest Canadian* in a national poll conducted by the Canadian Broadcasting Corporation in 2004. He was born in Scotland in 1904 but moved to Canada with his family when he was young. On becoming a Baptist minister, he was strongly influenced by the social gospel tradition, which combined Christian religious values with those of social reform (Ives, 2011). He became Premier of the province of Saskatchewan in 1944, and his party led the development of provincial healthcare in 1962, which was subsequently adopted nationwide. It was this tradition of so-called prairie socialism which formed the backdrop to the development of the baby-boomers (Savage, 2019). This caring for others, especially those most in need, was part of their identity, of which they were proud. Building upon this tradition, Pierre Trudeau, who became Prime Minister of Canada in 1968, championed what he termed the 'just society', which would ensure that 'No one in the society should be entitled to superfluous or luxury goods until the essentials of life are made available to everyone' (Trudeau, 1998). This was the boomers' Canada. The socialized healthcare system was part of their identity as Canadians and differentiated them from the United States, which was considered uncivilized.

However, their communitarian ethic was mixed with an individualistic ethic of success through hard work and personal ambition. The traditional class divide apparent in Britain is more concealed in Canada. A survey in 2023 found that only a minority identified as working class, while over 40% identified as middle class (Angus Reid, 2023). It was this belief in individual achievement that balanced support for healthcare with strong support for healthy lifestyles. You had a responsibility to be healthy and to lead a healthy life.

Work/non-work could be considered a thema that pervades the social representation of health and illness. Among the older Scottish residents, the ability to work and to work hard was intrinsic to their identity and health. Loss of work was not simply measured in economic terms but also in psychological terms. Additionally, refusal to work or poor working practices were reflective of poor moral character. Among the Canadian baby-boomers, health was something you had to work at. It was not something that was readily given, but as good Canadians, you were responsible for your health. While they were proud of the Canadian healthcare system, it was seen as being for those who were not responsible for any health problems they had. You had a duty to look after yourself.

Social representations not only develop from everyday social interaction but also from engagement with literature and the media. The narrative psychologist Sarbin (1997) argued that stories, whether read or heard, can provide the plot structures for one's own self-narratives. This is known as the Quixotic principle, named after Cervantes' *Don Quixote* (Pérez-Álvarez, 2006). Sarbin went on to argue that it is not just written stories but broader cultural myths that can provide a framework for our narrative identity. He cited the example of American cowboys and frontiersmen, who have been written about in many novels and portrayed in films, as providing the imaginings for contemporary adventurers. Kleinfeld (2012) has similarly commented on the power of the frontier myth in shaping the identity of some people who have moved to live in Alaska. While Scottish literature has often featured hardship and the value of hard work (e.g., Grassic Gibbon, 2006), Canadian literature was often imbued with images of the creation of a new and fairer world. These images pervade the identity of the older Scottish residents and the Canadian baby-boomers and are conveyed in their social representations. However, these societies are changing and new forms of literature and the arts has arisen to reflect these changes. Despite these changes, identities and social representations can draw on older ideas and experiences. For example, in his poetry, the Scottish poet Sorley MacLean (2014) writes about how ancient stories of defeat and loss still echo in the lives of Scottish people today: 'I go westward in the Desert | with my shame on my shoulders, | that I was made a laughing stock | since I was as my people were' while contemporary Canadian literature will often dwell on the historic treatment of indigenous peoples (Jackson, 2023). With the growth of technology, social representations may also increasingly draw upon future as well as past experiences as represented in new literary forms.

References

Angus Reid. (2023). *Canadians and class.* Angus Reid. 2023.09.21_Great_Canadian_Class_Survey.pdf. http://www.angusreid.org

Browne, A. (2004). Healthcare reform in Canada: The Romanow report. *Cambridge Quarterly of Healthcare Ethics, 13*(3), 221–225.

Caillaud, S., Kalampalikis, N., & Doumergue, M. (2022). Designing focus groups. In U. Flick (Ed.), *The SAGE handbook of qualitative research design* (pp. 684–699). Sage.

Cornelissen, L. (2021). *Religiosity in Canada and its evolution from 1985 to 2019.* Statistics Canada.

Cox, L. S., Mason, P. A., & Bagley, M. C. (2014). Understanding ageing: Biological and social perspectives. In A. Walker (Eds.), *The new science of ageing* (pp. 25–75). Policy.

Crow, G. (2021). In search of role models of successful academic retirement. *Contemporary Social Science, 16*(5), 604–617.
Eaton, D. H. (2013). The economists of the reformation: An overview of reformation teaching concerning work, wealth and interest. *SAGE Open, 3*(3).
Erikson, J. M. (1997). Preface. In *The life cycle completed: Extended edition* (pp. 1–9). W.W. Norton.
Fairhurst, E. (1998). 'Growing old gracefully' as opposed to 'mutton dressed as lamb': The social construction of recognising older women. In S. Nettleton & J. Watson (Eds.), *The body in everyday life* (pp. 258–275). Routledge.
Flick, U. (1992). Triangulation revisited: Strategy of validation or alternative? *Journal for the Theory of Social Behaviour, 22*(2), 175–192.
Flick, U., Fischer, C., Neuber, A., Schwartz, F. W., & Walter, U. (2003). Health in the context of growing old: Social representations of health. *Journal of Health Psychology, 8*(5), 539–556.
Flick, U., Fischer, C., Schwartz, F. W., & Walter, U. (2002). Social representations of health held by health professionals: The case of general practitioners and home-care nurses. *Social Science Information, 41*(4), 581–602.
Foot, D. K. (1999). *Boom, bust and echo 2000: Profiting from the demographic shift in the new millennium*. Macfarlane Walter & Ross.
Grassic Gibbon, L. (2006). *A scots quair. The mearns trilogy*. Polygon.
Hepworth, M. (2000). *Stories of ageing*. Open University Press.
Herzlich, C. (1973). *Health and illness: A social psychological analysis*. Academic Press. (Original: *Santé et Maladie: Analyse d'une Réprésentation Sociale*. Paris: Mouton, 1969).
Ives, A. (2011). Christians on the left: The importance of the social gospel in the Canadian social democratic tradition. *Revue LISA/LISA e-Journal, 9*(1), 188–204.
Jackson, S. -N. (2023). Canadian fictions. *Canadian Literature, 252*, 9–14.
Just, D. (2014). The invention of work in modernity: Hegel, Marx, and Weber. *Journal of Historical Sociology, 30*(2), 435–456.
Kampmann, S. (2015). Visual aging studies: Exploring images of aging in art history and other disciplines. *Age Culture Humanities, 2*, 279–290.
Kaufman, J. R. (1994). The social construction of frailty: An anthropological perspective. *Journal of Aging Studies, 8*(1), 45–58.
Kleinfeld, J. (2012). *The frontier romance: Environment, culture, and Alaska identity*. University of Alaska Press.
Lalonde, M. (1974). *A new perspective on the health of Canadians*. Government of Canada.
MacLean, S. (2014). *Hallaig and other poems*. Polygon.
Murray, M., Pullman, D., & Rodgers, T. H. (2003). Social representations of health and illness among baby-boomers in Eastern Canada. *Journal of Health Psychology, 8*(5), 485–499.

Murray, M., Pullman, D., Turner, L., & Simpson, E. (1999). *Norms and narratives: Beliefs regarding health in an ageing population, research proposal.* Social Science and Humanities Research Council.

Murray, M., & Rodgers, T. H. (2002). *Atlantic Canada baby-boomers' representations of health, illness and aging. Norms and Narratives, Research Report II.* Memorial University.

Pérez-Álvarez, M. (2006). The psychology of Don Quixote. *Psychology in Spain, 10*, 17–27.

Potvin, L., & Jones, C. M. (2011). Twenty-five years after the Ottawa Charter: The critical role of health promotion for public health. *Canadian Journal of Public Health, 102*(4), 244–248.

Romanow, R. (2002). *Building on values: The future of healthcare in Canada.* Government of Canada.

Sarbin, T. R. (1997). The poetics of identity. *Theory & Psychology, 7*(1), 67–82.

Savage, L. (2019). Tommy Douglas, Canada's Great Prairie socialist, wasn't always so beloved. *The Jacobin.* Tommy Douglas, Canada's Great Prairie Socialist, Wasn't Always so Beloved. http://www.Jacobin.com.

Smith, R. (2009). Religion, the Scottish work ethic and the spirit of enterprise. *Entrepreneurship and Innovation, 10*(2), 111–124.

Tiedemann, M. (2019). *The Canada health act: An overview.* Library of Parliament.

Trudeau, P. E. (1998). *The essential trudeau* (R. Graham, Ed.). McClelland & Stewart.

Vernon, J. A., Williams, J. A., Phillips, T., & Wilson, J. (1991). Media stereotyping: A comparison of the way elderly women and men are portrayed on primetime television. *Journal of Women and Aging, 2*(4), 55–68.

Von Hülsen-Esch, A. (2022). *Cultural perspectives on aging: A different approach to old age and aging.* De Gruyter.

Walker, A. (Ed.). (2014). *The new science of ageing.* Policy.

Waltz, M., & Gran, B. K. (2017). Portrayal of older adults in popular television shows. In G. Joseph (Ed.), *Diverse perspectives on aging in a changing world* (pp. 24–37). Routledge.

Warren, L. (2018). Representing self-representing aging. In A. Walker (Ed.), *The new dynamics of ageing* (Vol. 2, pp. 219–242). Polity.

WHO. (1986). *The Ottawa Charter for health promotion.* WHO Regional Office for Europe.

Williams, R. (1983). Concepts of health: An analysis of lay logic. *Sociology, 17*(2), 185–205.

Williams, R. (1990). *A protestant legacy: Attitudes to death and illness among older Aberdonians.* Clarendon Press.

PART III

Social Representations and Change

CHAPTER 8

Stability and Change

Social representations of health and illness are dynamic social constructions in a particular time and place. They not only impose themselves on us, but they can also be challenged and transformed in everyday social interaction. This chapter considers these change processes. It focuses on the role of the minority in initiating change. It also returns to the concept of narrative as a means of conceptualizing the change process.

8.1 Stability of Social Representations

In the previous chapters, we have explored how communities develop social representations of health and illness. We emphasized that these representations are not merely cognitive constructions but rather social psychological phenomena that reflect the character of the communities' social engagement. As Jovchelovitch (2007) argued: 'Rather than define these systems of knowledge as ignorance, distortion and error, they are understood as the practical means of a community to express itself, its identity and way of life' (p. 165).

Social representations are resistant to change because they are intimately related to how we define ourselves, and they also reflect certain power dynamics in society. Forming social representations helps to define a group, promote in-group solidarity and defend group members from out-group threats. Consider the case of the Ebola virus, which is deadly if

M. Murray, *Social Representations, Health and Illness*,
https://doi.org/10.1007/978-3-031-98494-5_8

contracted. Interviews conducted in Britain about this virus found that most lay people portrayed it as an African disease that they were very unlikely to contract. As one woman said: 'It just seemed like one of those mythical diseases, sort of thing, science fiction like thing, that happens in places like Africa and underdeveloped countries and doesn't come here' (Joffe & Haarhoff, 2002, p. 965). By clearly characterizing the disease in fantastical terms, the lay public was symbolically protecting itself from this outside threat while continuing to go about their everyday lives. In a comparable study of social representations of AIDS in Zambia (Joffe & Bettega, 2004), it was found that young residents distanced themselves from the risk of the disease by representing it as originating in Western society and in deviant sexual and scientific practices. These findings highlighted the challenge of encouraging young people to take personal action to protect themselves against AIDS, since it was represented as something alien to their society.

In addition, the stability of social representations is maintained by certain power dynamics. Negura et al. (2020) argued that one way to conceptualize these power dynamics was to consider power as operating at the three different levels proposed by Jodelet (2012). At the trans-subjective level, the power of dominant groups is legitimized through social representations, which are anchored in themata, ideologies and social norms. At the inter-subjective level, power operates through the type of communication imposed by social representations. Finally, at the subjective level, social representations enable the internalization of power. This approach conceptualizes how power is internalized and results in the process of self-discipline.

Hegemonic social representations, which operate at the trans-subjective level, can serve to legitimize social inequalities in health and illness and promote individualistic explanations. These, in turn, can be reinforced through health professionals ignoring the broader social circumstances of people's lives. Legislation to address the social determinants of health and illness through various measures can be hindered by the emphasis on promoting the infrastructure of clinical/technological medicine. At the inter-subjective level, the associated health professionals can also act to promote this approach to healthcare. The power of medicine is buttressed by ancient social representations of the witch-doctor or shaman, which provide them with greater power than that afforded by biomedicine. At the subjective level, this archaic representation is internalized such that the patient treats the doctor with respect and reverence, which remains high despite various controversies (Kmietovicz, 2002).

It is also important to bear in mind the concept of cognitive polyphasia, whereby a group or community can manage different social representations. For example, the community can have both traditional as well as biomedical conceptions of health and illness. The dominance of particular social representations can be challenged depending on circumstances. However, since traditional social representations will have developed over a sustained period, they are resistant to change. Jovchelovitch and Gervais (1999), in their study of the different social representations of health held by people of Chinese heritage in London, showed how these representations enabled them to sustain and defend their community identity. They could hold both Western and Chinese representations of health in tandem as a means of maintaining their ethnic identity in Western society.

An example of the resistance to health-related change was exhibited in a study of a cancer prevention campaign in a working-class community in America (Balshem, 1990). This study was conducted in two communities in Philadelphia during the early 1980s. It had been found that these communities had high rates of cancer, so it was decided to launch a standard health education campaign advising residents of the communities to quit smoking and improve their diet. However, the residents were resistant to this message, identifying industrial pollution as the major cause of the disease. The medical professionals saw the residents as misguided and as being responsible for the high rate of cancer, while the residents saw the physicians as arrogant and controlling. Balshem highlighted the distinction between the scientific representation of cancer held by the physicians and educators and the more localized social representation of the disease rooted in the everyday experience of the residents. Although the medical professionals had the power and status, they were not able to impose their view, which was seen as unrealistic and as not fitting with the local residents' social representations of the disease.

Further, social representations of health are concretized in social institutions and organizations as well as their physical manifestations in buildings (Howarth et al., 2004). These physical manifestations reinforce the hegemonic social representation of disease as a solely biomedical phenomenon.

The historic character of social representations of illness may remain hidden but is revealed at times of crisis, when supposedly arcane social representations are brought to the fore as a means of making sense of a crisis. For example, the recent outbreak of various disease pandemics brought forward various older ideas about the organization of society. In the case of HIV/AIDS, it was ideas about appropriate sexual behaviour and divine retribution for supposed deviancy. In the case of COVID-19, it was ancient ideas about the 'yellow peril' or threats to Western civilization from Chinese practices.

In the political domain, these ancient ideas also come to the fore at times of crisis. In *The Eighteenth Brumaire of Louis Bonaparte*, Marx (1852) emphasized that history hangs heavily over our everyday lives:

> Men make their own history, but they do not make it as they please; they do not make it under self-selected circumstances, but under circumstances existing already, given and transmitted from the past. The tradition of all dead generations weighs like a nightmare on the brains of the living. And just as they seem to be occupied with revolutionizing themselves and things, creating something that did not exist before, precisely in such epochs of revolutionary crisis, they anxiously conjure up the spirits of the past to their service, borrowing from them names, battle slogans, and costumes in order to present this new scene in world history in time-honoured disguise and borrowed language (Marx, 1852, p. 5).

More recently, a similar point was made by Caroline Howarth and colleagues in detailing the role of the past in constraining changes in social representations of health and illness.

> We can, and do, change our representations, but always within the possibilities and constraints of past and present. In presenting, reflecting and enacting how we think about health and illness within the context to the everyday, for example, we may become self-conscious of our own social representations. Consequently, the act of representing the social world carries with it the possibility for critique and transformation (Howarth et al., 2004, p. 237).

It is this potential for critique and transformation that offers opportunities for activities designed to promote health.

8.2 Social Representations and Change

Social representations are dynamic social psychological processes that contain tensions and contradictions. As such, they present 'possibilities for communication, negotiation, resistance, innovation and transformation' (Howarth, 2006, p. 68). Resistance to oppressive social representations can take place at different levels, from the individual through to the societal (cf. Doise, 1986). The individual, through his or her position in society, can publicly challenge certain social representations but is stymied in developing change until he or she begins to gain the support of others. Moscovici was particularly enthused by the power of the minority in challenging and transforming dominant social representations.

While social representations exert an 'irresistible force' (Moscovici, 1984, p. 9) on our understanding of the world, there remains the possibility of subverting and challenging these. The trend towards constancy in social representations is balanced by a trend towards transformation and change. As Himmelweit (1990) argued, change is ever-present in society due to a variety of factors, including 'disaffection of individual members, minority influences, conflicting values within the complex subsystems of a society, outside events, changes in the economy, or the consequences of the introduction of new technologies' (p. 24).

This focus on change was taken up by Howarth et al. (2013) who argued that societal psychology is concerned with 'the contexts which promote or inhibit social and societal change' (p. 364). Furthermore, they argued that social change has largely been concerned with change at the individual and group level, whereas societal psychology 'examines change within a broader political context, and incorporates change at the level of communities, organisations, governments, and international networks' (p. 365). They argued that societal psychology offers opportunities to examine the work of community groups instituting change, the processes of change itself, and the impact of societal psychological knowledge.

In her discussion of the legacy of Moscovici, Jovchelovitch (2019) detailed the resistance of social representations to change.

> Social representations are the ideas we live by and sometimes will die for. Created and transformed through communication in the public sphere, they go around in histories and stories, cultures and generations. They change, but do not go away (p. 165).

However, this does not mean that we should accept this resistance to change. She continued:

> Moscovici did not seek to rehabilitate common sense in order to describe it and accept it; I think it is fair to say that his project was one of *understanding*, and therefore of transformation (p. 167).

She argued that the debate about change can be traced back to the differences in the approaches of Plato and Socrates. After the death of Socrates, Plato despaired and denounced the views of the general public, instead arguing that only outside of it was it possible to grasp the higher truth. Socrates, on the other hand, positioned himself within the *polis*: 'Socrates walked the city wanting to help his fellow *polis* human beings to find the truth in their *doxa* (opinion)' (Jovchelovitch, 2019, p. 169). It is in this process of dialogue that 'interlocutors worked together to move forward an understanding of the world' (Jovchelovitch, 2019, p. 169). In the same way, it was through dialogue and debate that Moscovici sought not only understanding but transformation.

From the outset, Moscovici was concerned not only with understanding common sense but also with transforming it. He criticized both the educative approach of the Enlightenment and the propaganda of the Leninists both of which he considered too one-sided. Instead, he was concerned with how you can work with collectives to transform repressive social representations. As Howarth (2006) argued: 'Resistance is simultaneously a social and psychological possibility. It is through the very process of social re-presentation that meanings become ambiguous, hybrid and contested. This then presents the possibilities of dialogue, debate and conflict' (p. 77). The challenge is to explore processes of change.

One way of considering the social change cycle, suggested by Castro and Mouro (2011), is that it operates through three stages: the emergence stage, in which innovative ideas are put forward, often by a minority, and begin to gain support. This is followed by the institutional stage, when the ideas are taken up and formulated into policy. Then there is the generalization stage, when the policy becomes translated into locally agreed ways of acting. Here, we will consider how the minority can begin to exert change in social representations of health and illness.

8.2.1 Power of Minorities

Minorities have an important role to play in initiating challenge and change. The early research by Asch (1951) was designed to demonstrate that the majority view within a group led to the minority conforming. In his experiment, the participants were asked to assess the comparative lengths of a series of lines. The majority of the groups were collaborators of Asch, who asserted that certain lines were of the same length. The minority in the group conformed to the view of the group majority, which Asch argued demonstrated the power of the majority. However, Moscovici ([1976] 2008) argued that this research experiment was taken out of the larger social context. When this context was considered, the majority in the group were actually a minority in the broader social world, while the minority were in accord with the real-world majority. Thus, the experiment was a demonstration of the power of the minority.

Moscovici ([1976] 2008) further distinguished between compliance and conversion. Compliance is the process where the participants publicly conform to the majority view but privately reject it. This was the case for many in Asch's experiments. Conversion is when the participants both publicly and privately conform. This is the process by which the minority convinces the majority that their views are correct. This is the internalization of the minority viewpoint, which occurs in different situations.

Four factors were identified as important in achieving conversion. These are *behavioural style, style of thinking, flexibility* and *identification. Behavioural style* refers to the overt behaviour of the minority group who are engaged in promoting conversion. This style has four components:

1. Consistency, whereby the minority continues to express a certain view.
2. Confidence, whereby the minority expresses strength in their opinion.
3. Unbiased, which is concerned with how the minority appears, aims to express an impartial and balanced viewpoint.
4. Resistance whereby the minority resists social pressure to renounce their view.

These four components are interlinked, but the most important is consistency. The reason for this is that the majority will begin to reassess their own viewpoint if the minority consistently expresses a contrary position. The consistency of the minority presents an image that the minority is committed to their viewpoint and is not simply expressing a fleeting opinion. Confronted by a minority who is self-confident and resistant to change, the majority begins to reassess the validity of their view. The consistency of the minority begins to disrupt established norms and sows seeds of doubt among the majority.

Style of thinking is the process whereby the minority encourages the majority to grasp pro and counter-arguments. When the majority can grasp opposing points of view, they are more receptive to change (Nemeth, 1995). *Flexibility* is concerned with the extent of flexibility in how the message is presented. Although consistency is important, its impact depends upon how it is perceived by others. If it is perceived as being inflexible and dogmatic, it is more likely to be rejected. However, if there is evidence of flexibility and the minority is seen to be taking the views of others into consideration, then the minority view is more likely to be accepted. However, if the minority is too flexible, it would give the impression of a lack of consistency, and the majority may begin to doubt the commitment of the minority. *Identification* is the extent to which the majority can identify with the minority. If the minority is viewed as similar, then the majority is more accepting of their views, while if the minority is viewed as dissimilar, their impact is less.

In the political sphere, minorities have historically played a key role in initiating change in society. Moscovici (1979) conducted a detailed examination of literary texts by famous dissidents, including Aleksandr Solzhenitsyn and Andrei Sakharov, to tease out the processes involved in minority influence (Moscovici & Marková, 2000, p. 267). He argued that social representations underlie behavioural style. It was the promotion of polemical social representations that enabled the minority to influence the majority. Solzhenitsyn and Sakharov shared their social representation of repression and action with the majority. It was then through their consistent and courageous opposition to repression that they began to have an impact.

Minorities can exert substantial influence not only by using the four strategies outlined by Moscovici but also by displaying courage and self-sacrifice. This feature is evident in the autobiographical accounts written by political activists. In her analysis of the autobiographies of nineteenth- and twentieth-century women political activists, Watson (1999) described their accounts as rhetorical narratives. They were not written as a form of self-promotion but to encourage the reader to join the bigger cause of fighting for social change. As she said, 'They were written to create an audience for their causes; by offering an appealing image of womanhood through enacting in their own lives, they work to generate new support and allegiance among the formerly uncommitted' (p. 5). They aimed to promote identification with themselves and their cause. They also strove to achieve this through a consistent message and apparent self-sacrifice. They presented their message not in a dogmatic fashion but with flexibility and with little concern for their own survival.

Blood sacrifice has frequently been used by revolutionaries to emphasize the momentous nature of the change they were proposing. Karl Liebknecht, the German Marxist leader who had led an unsuccessful revolt in 1919, said of his followers: 'They have shed blood for a holy cause, which has thus been sanctified. And from every drop of their blood, this seed of dragons for the winners of today, will rise the fallen Avenger' (Fallon, 2016). This idea of blood sacrifice has been a frequent theme in many revolutionary and religious writings.

In her study of the narrative character of the Christian gospels, Bond (2000) described how they were written to attract people to this new religion. The emphasis in these gospels was on self-sacrifice, which was epitomized in the death of Christ. Reed (2017), in his study of political activists in Nicaragua, found that such religious stories of self-sacrifice and redemption were interwoven into their discussions of political change. The case of Socrates is similar. He accepted the hemlock and died to illustrate to his followers his commitment to his ideas and to serve as an example for them to follow those ideas.

Another important change factor was the articulation of a clear change narrative. A study of the autobiographical accounts of two Scottish community activists demonstrated that their rhetorical character aimed not at self-aggrandizement but rather to highlight that things did not have to be as they were (Murray, 2020). The message was to offer a vision of change with which people could identify. As Selbin (2010) argued: 'Revolution, rebellion and acts of resistance do not occur without the articulation of compelling stories that enable and empower people who seek to change the material and ideological conditions of their lives' (p. 194). It is through promoting this vision of change that political and other leaders can convince people that the system is not impermeable. They can begin to challenge the dominance of repressive hegemonic social representations.

The two Scottish activists worked to offer a future narrative of change in disadvantaged communities. As such, they were challenging the internalization of the negative social representation of those communities and the acceptance of a lack of resources and healthcare. It was through engagement in various activities that the residents became aware of their talents and strengths. This narrative of hope is core to the polemical social representation and offers a rallying point for social change. Their accounts also raised the challenge experienced by the community activists of self-sacrifice versus personal aggrandizement.

An understanding of the power of minorities must also take into consideration the broader socio-cultural context and the extent to which opposition is allowed. These women were active in the 1980s, which was a period of sustained industrial strife in Britain. It was within this context that they were able to involve communities in campaigns for better conditions. Forty years later, with the rise of neo-liberalism, the sense of community is not so clear-cut. There has been much research on the decline in social capital in the West (Putnam, 2000). Specific research on the impact of neo-liberalism has shown that the more neo-liberal people perceive their society to be, the lesser their sense of connection to others and the greater their sense of competition (Becker et al., 2021). This would suggest that the minority group will find it more difficult to garner support at this time. However, the greater the perceived social and economic injustice, the more likely the minority are to gather support (Power, 2018).

8.2.2 *Impact of Minority on Health Action*

In the health arena, certain organized minority groups within society can subvert hegemonic social representations. Using biographical interviews, we explored the life histories of a sample of community health workers (Murray & Ziegler, 2015). The everyday activities of these workers focused on encouraging residents to become more actively involved in their community and to take action to address health inequalities. In this study, a sample of twelve community workers was interviewed about their lives and their work. A central theme in their recollections was their commitment to social justice and community empowerment. This was expressed by one worker:

> I used to be very, very proud of this job, really proud to be part of this, and I do, it meets my belief that we should challenge health inequalities; we should challenge social inequality in general. I meet my beliefs so much, 'cos, you know, I'd love to imagine that there was some impact, and I'd like to be meeting people. I'd really like to be meeting people who have got, erm, challenging lives and offer, you know, a little bit of change. And I also love, erm, the fact that we can work in a slightly, well in a very, we have been able to work in a very creative way (p. 342).

The community workers were frustrated by the social representation of the community in which they worked, which portrayed it as being home to people who were feckless and brought disadvantage upon themselves. They were also frustrated that many of the residents had internalized this social representation and thought of themselves and their neighbours as worthless, as though they had been rejected and forgotten by authority. The community workers aimed to work with the residents to challenge this negative self-social representation and, in turn, to challenge the one held by authority.

Several of the community workers proudly recalled the socialist heritage of their families, which emphasized support for the weakest and cooperation with neighbours. In terms of behavioural style, the workers emphasized the importance of being consistent in their message and of continuing to pursue an empowerment agenda in their work, despite encountering many setbacks:

> Our job is to be very consistent always be ready and keep providing information, because one time you provide information and help if you're just there, you're available which is another part of the job, being available I think, erm, perhaps somebody will get on the cycle of change, you know, if it's as simple as that, if they get that motivator or, erm. But you've got to be around, you know, you can't withdraw that that's really hard for services, 'cos obviously if you don't get results in a six-week period, you know, 'it's not working, I've got finite resources. I've got to deal with other things (p. 342–343).

In terms of identification with the community, the community workers spoke about the importance of self-denial. As one worker said, it was important to 'give a bit of yourself'. This took place over an extended period during which they shared experiences with the residents and gained their confidence. One worker described the need to get the community 'under your skin'. He continued, 'Unless you sort of feel a little bit like you're part of the community, you're never going to truly understand what people in that area want' (p. 343).

It was through consistent, dedicated work in the community that the worker gained the confidence of the residents and was able to work with them to begin collectively challenging the negative representations of the community. Together, these studies illustrate the role of the minority in challenging particular negative social representations and moving from agitation through to policy change, resulting in increased resources for the community.

8.2.3 Groupwork

Groups provide an opportunity for participants to reflect on dominant negative social representations of health and other issues. As such, they can be considered to act as a minority in opposition to the apparent majority view outside the group. An example is the self-help group for people who are affected by certain health problems. Krause (2003) conducted a study in Chile of a self-help group for people with inflammatory bowel disease. In that study, 19 people diagnosed with the disease met on a weekly basis to discuss the disease and ways of dealing with it. At the outset, the participants had a negative representation of the disease, which was seen as negatively impacting all aspects of their lives. Several of the participants were reluctant to accept the diagnosis as a means of protecting themselves. Others were consigned to a fatalistic acceptance of the negative consequences. Throughout the group meetings, the participants sought further information about the disease as well as reassurance from other participants that, although it was a chronic disease, it was possible to live with it. At the close of the self-help group meetings, the participants had a more positive representation of the disease. It was something that they could live with. The participants saw themselves as less ill and as less handicapped. There were also reduced levels of shame and a greater ability to talk about the disease.

Another example of the impact of participation in groups on social representations of ageing was apparent in the study of reading groups by older people (Hubble & Tew, 2013). In this study, which was conducted in London between 2009 and 2012, eight reading groups, totalling 80 older participants, met monthly to read and discuss nine novels that featured older people. The participants kept diaries to record their initial impressions after reading each of these novels and their impressions after the group discussion. An important aspect of these reading groups was the opportunity for the participants to not only reflect on the content of the novels but also on how their portrayal of older people connected with their own life experiences. In reading alone, the participants began the process of questioning the dominant negative representation of ageing that was often central to many of the novels. Their views were then discussed further in the reading groups.

Through reading and reflecting on the novels with others in the groups, they were able to challenge the dominant social representation of ageing as one of inevitable decline. This was something that Nick Hubble and Philip Tew placed in a broader historical context of post-war capitalism, which positioned older people as not being potentially productive to the system and so could be consigned to institutions to live out their last days. Admittedly, the participants in this study were middle-class and educated and resisted this social exclusion. As one said about retirement: 'I'm having a whale of a time' (p. 126). They also noted how representations of ageing had changed in their lifetime. One participant reflected on the increase in intergenerational activity: 'The present young and middle aged seem to share inside as well as outside the home to a greater extent' (p. 81).

The study expanded our understanding of social representations of ageing as something that is polyphasic, such that the hegemonic representation of decline can be contested. However, the social isolation of older people makes this contestation more difficult. The internalization of this negative representation reduces the agency of the older person. This was something that was challenged in other participatory projects.

These reading groups were based on discussing a book that group members had previously read. An alternative format is to promote reading aloud from the book at the group meetings. This is the format favoured by The Reader network of reading groups in Britain (Billington, 2016). These and other groups are not designed to address specific health issues but to promote reading for pleasure. They also promote the value of being with other group members and provide an opportunity for the group to reflect on the portrayal of health and other issues by different authors. Billington has argued that the very act of reading allows participants to articulate their own experiences and to begin questioning dominant social representations.

In a small study conducted in the English Midlands in the 2010s, the impact of participation in such reading groups was explored (Seymour & Murray, 2016). In this study, a group of residents from a nursing home met on a weekly basis to read and discuss a selection of poems. Thematic analysis of the group discussions revealed a primary and recurrent theme of life as a process of change. In doing so, they were reflecting on the traditional representation of ageing as one of decline and counter-posing an alternative view of older age as being an opportunity to explore new approaches and activities. As one woman said: 'I think we renew ourselves in the way we think, you see' (p. 197).

8.2.4 Community Action

Another important focus has been on the work of minorities within disadvantaged communities to promote health and wellbeing. The past 50 years have witnessed the development of many community-based approaches to promoting health. These approaches combine popular education with community-based research and social action to address specific health issues and inequalities. In this action, the community activist works with residents to identify a concern of the community and to develop and implement a plan to address that issue. These are iterative processes, such that the initial community dialogue proceeds to the development and implementation of an action plan and then returns to a review and dialogue.

This community approach to health action has been influenced by the critical literacy work of Paulo Freire (1921–1997). His original work came to prominence at a time of sustained political oppression in Brazil (Freire, [1968] 1997). He argued at that time that critical education could play an important role in transforming society. The aim of this form of education was *conscientização,* which has been translated by Myra Bergman Ramos as 'learning to perceive social, political, and economic contradictions, and to take action against oppressive elements of reality' (Freire, [1968] 1997, p. 17). Freire's pedagogy of the oppressed was the process by which people begin to engage in the process of critical reflection and action. As he said:

> To surmount the situation of oppression, people must first critically recognise its causes, so it is through transforming action they can create a new situation, one which makes possible the pursuit of a new humanity (p. 29).

In developing this approach, Freire was, in some ways, akin to Moscovici in his reluctance to impose change from above through propaganda, but rather by dialogue and debate within a particular community. He was guided by a philosophy to treat other people as Subjects rather than Objects, as people who can actively play a role in historical processes rather than be acted upon by others.

His work is detailed in several books, including the classic *Pedagogy of the Oppressed* (Freire, [1968] 1997). In this work, he emphasized the importance of collaborative work:

> This person does not consider himself or herself the proprietor of history or of all people, or the liberator of the oppressed; but he or she does commit himself or herself, within history, to fight at their side (p. 21).

The basic Freirean approach is encapsulated in the 'diagnosis-action-reflection' cycle, in which the external change agent works with the oppressed community to increase their awareness of their circumstances and contribute to collective mobilization to transform their oppressive social conditions. This approach has formed the basis of community health psychology (Campbell & Murray, 2004; Campbell & Cornish, 2014).

Community health psychology is an approach that takes the social representations of a community as the starting point for its practice. However, it combines this with an awareness of broader structural inequalities that persist in society and a commitment to social transformation. Furthermore, rather than imposing a change framework on the community, it begins by grasping the issues that the community members consider problematic and works with them to formulate a change strategy.

However, this community-level approach must also take into consideration the changing socio-political situation. Nolas (2014) reassessed the contribution of Freire and suggested that we explore his later writings. She characterized his *Pedagogy of the Oppressed* (Freire, [1968] 1997) as providing a 'map' detailing the character of the change process. She termed his description of the change process in his later writing in the *Pedagogy of Hope* (Freire, 1994) as a 'journey' which detailed the 'lived experience of the everyday practice of collective action which relies on the enmeshment of a range of cognitive, emotional and practical influences' (p. 127). Campbell (2014) concluded that there was a need for more flexibility in its application. Specifically, she argued that global finance capitalism is ever more ingenuous in its reach and has to be combatted in various ways. Also, the increasing awareness of inter-sectionality requires community activists to broaden their remit from purely economic issues.

The lack of attention to the details of the journey in some community psychology is compounded by the demands of academic research organization which are based on short-term funding and quick results. This is especially the case in psychology, which has been dominated by experimental research designs. Other social science disciplines provide greater opportunities to present interim results and details of the processes of change.

Another important factor is the almost medicalization of community health action. There is sometimes an expectation that the intervention can lead to a 'cure' in a short-term process. Contrast that with the management of chronic illness, which is long-term support rather than a cure. Adopting this approach emphasizes the need for ongoing support for participatory interventions. Also, rather than imposing an agenda on the community, it means working with it as part of the process of social and community enhancement. Consider again the work of the community and political activists. This places a moral or ethical frame on participatory research. It is something designed for working with rather than working on (Murray et al., 2004). In this sense, it can learn from liberation psychology, which was developed in Latin America by Ignacio Martin-Baro from the work of the liberation theology of Gustavo Gutierrez (Murray, 2012). He argued for the need to take the 'preferential option for the poor' if we are to enhance the broader health of society. The poor are not simply those with limited income but rather those who are lacking in power and are oppressed in various ways.

In their discussion of transformation in a Brazilian community, Guareschi and Jovchelovitch (2004) proposed an approach similar to that earlier described by Castro and Mauro. They identified three phases in the transformation process: diagnosis, intervention and critical reflexivity. Diagnosis is the process of working with the community to grasp their representations and practices. Intervention is the process of change and is based upon the conviction that 'the health of the poor depends on the political capacity of grassroots to articulate demands and produce pressure from below' (p. 316). Critical reflexivity is the process of reflecting on and developing alternatives: 'Reality is a field of open possibilities and rather than describing it, the task of knowledge is to identify critically which alternatives can transform it' (p. 317).

Social representations develop in certain times and places, such that community interventions must consider the changing circumstances in which people live and work. Community development needs to take into consideration the continuing social inequalities in society. Community action does not provide a one-off solution to the health problems facing people, but it is part of the broader process of change. There is the danger, when working at the community level, of evading consideration of the broader social inequalities and instead turning to a form of collective victim-blaming (Murray, 2012). We need to consider the material and symbolic circumstances within which we work. At the outset, we commented on Moscovici's engagement with Marxist theory, where he recognized the importance of material circumstances. While we can engage in campaigns at the community and societal level to challenge oppressive social representations, this also requires an awareness of the constraints of economic factors (Murray & Campbell, 2003).

A major challenge in these community projects is their potential to lead to sustained change. As was emphasized at the outset, the aim is not a total solution to the problem but rather a step on the road. Community health action is not the panacea but rather part of a broader process of social transformation.

8.3 Community Arts

Community arts is an approach to working with groups and communities in a collaborative manner to develop a range of creative activities and enhance health and well-being (Casey & Murray, 2022). Underlying this approach is a commitment to cultural democracy, which Webster and Buglass (2005) defined as a way to:

> promote the Arts in a way that is accessible, where all communities are valued, and where everyone has an opportunity to take a part. [This] would be a democracy in the real sense of the word, full of discussion, action and vibrancy. A culture made up of many voices, defined and representing all cultures and communities (p. 21).

Community arts is both inwardly satisfying to the community and outwardly challenging to various forms of social exclusion and oppression. As Webster and Buglass (2005) continued:

> [A] participatory arts activity would not only give people the understanding and knowledge to undertake arts activities, but [. . .] this process would give them insight into the nature of the oppressive ways in which society functions and give them the tools to do something about it (p. 9).

It is an approach that has a long heritage, drawing upon a number of theoretical orientations, either implicitly or explicitly. Several community arts projects illustrate how they can challenge certain oppressive social representations.

Central to this process is the power of storytelling. It is through the development and exchange of stories that people can begin to grasp the content of social representations. As Jovchelovitch (2007) said:

> It is by telling stories that knowledge comes into life, and with it, the representations of the past, and the presentations of identity. Through the telling of stories, communities recall what has happened (social memory), put experience into sequence (humanisation of time), find explanations for what is going on (sense making) and play with the chain of events that shapes individual and social life (future making) (p. 82).

As mentioned in previous chapters, social representations are developed through social interaction but are also maintained through stories and songs. The power of stories to transform social representations is illustrated in a series of community arts projects.

8.3.1 Health and Safety

The fishing industry is extremely dangerous, with multiple injuries and deaths reported annually. The FISH Safety Foundation (2022) has estimated that, on average, each year 100,000 people die while engaged in activities related to commercial fishing. Attempts to improve safety in the industry have followed various methods, from improvements in vessel design to regulations about fishing and safety education. Since it is difficult to police fishing regulations, there have been serious attempts to advance safety education through programmes designed to 'professionalize' the industry, including training programmes and licensing procedures. However, these safety training programmes have tended to focus on changing the knowledge and attitudes of individual fish harvesters rather than working with communities.

In 1990, a community safety programme was developed in three fishing communities in the Canadian province of Newfoundland. The fishing industry in these communities was largely of the small-boat character, involving fish harvesters on small vessels that would fish within a limited distance from the shore. Interviews with a sample of fish harvesters, followed by a survey of a larger sample, confirmed the high rate of injury and their acceptance of accidents as an intrinsic part of the industry. Their social representation of the industry as intrinsically dangerous was rooted in a lengthy community history of generations of fishing, together with practical experience of the industry. However, somewhat similar to Blaxter's study of perceived causes of illness, the fish harvesters often took responsibility for accidents, although these were considered part of the job (Murray & Dolomount, 1994).

That study was followed by the development of a community safety programme (Murray & Tilley, 2006). This involved working with fish harvesters, family members and other community residents in the design of a series of creative activities. These included dramatic performances, social events, visual displays and school-based activities. The aim of the study was not to formally evaluate these projects but to explore the impact of sharing stories about accidents and safety within the communities.

Two issues were important here. The first was the challenge to the dominant social representation of accidents as being not only expected but also an unavoidable component of the industry. Another challenge was the acceptance of the dangers as being part of the masculine culture associated with the industry (Hearn et al., 2023). The alternative approach was to reflect upon who was responsible for accidents and how everyone in the community had a role to play in promoting safety.

The second issue was the form of community development. The project did not follow a straight line but evolved over several years and experienced many ups and downs. For example, a teacher in the local school in one community offered to write and produce a play about accidents at sea. During the week of the performance, there was a heavy snowstorm, and the play was rescheduled for several months later. However, when that revised date arrived, there was an industrial dispute, and the play was cancelled again. Then the teacher moved to another town. After some months of disruption, other community members offered to produce the play, which was eventually performed after many mishaps. This toing and froing is very much typical of community development work and requires a long-term approach. As Nolas (2014) noted, the work of community health psychologists requires 'a good deal of energy, creativity, imagination, resilience, nimble footwork, readiness, patience, perseverance, empathy, pain, reflexivity and many other personal and interpersonal qualities and experiences on all sides' (p. 27).

Hundreds of community residents participated in this project, and it was widely reported in the media. It presented a social representation of safety as the responsibility of the community. However, the intrinsic dangers of the fishing industry remained.

8.3.2 Healthy Ageing

As with people who have chronic health problems, older people also report frequent exclusion from social life. They report being excluded from many opportunities, made to feel like a burden on society, and generally treated with disrespect in everyday social interactions. This social and psychological exclusion is compounded by structural inequalities, such that many older people reside in neighbourhoods with limited facilities, a lack of accessible transport, poor housing quality and high levels of crime. These factors contribute to marginalization and social exclusion. This social exclusion is central to their social representation of ageing (Walker, 2014).

A qualitative study conducted among older residents of three cities in the UK detailed the social exclusion experienced by older people (Menezes et al., 2023). It was found that many older people reported becoming invisible to other city dwellers. For example, one older woman said: 'I've noticed in the last maybe what, certainly the last few years, I'm just 65 now, but you become invisible. You really do'. This exclusion from social opportunities leads to feelings of rejection and social inadequacy.

The *CALL-ME Study* consisted of the participatory development of a series of community projects with older residents living in disadvantaged areas of a city in northern England. One of these projects was a community arts initiative that was developed in an inner-city neighbourhood (Murray & Crummett, 2010). This initiative took place over a period of 18 months and involved a series of smaller arts projects that were developed with older residents under the guidance of community arts workers.

In the initial interviews and discussions with the participants, they clearly identified with their community, which they felt had been ignored and neglected. Most of the participants had lived in the neighbourhood for 40 years or more and recalled their changing experiences—from a time of hope and optimism to one of pessimism and resignation. The community was described in terms of limited opportunities and resources, as well as general neglect. This negative social representation of their community was augmented by what the residents felt others (both local government officials and other city residents) thought of their neighbourhood. One male resident said:

> We're a forgotten area and always have been. When you get the newsletter it's all about that end [neighbouring community], there's never anything about us. I think it's happened because they never give us anything, well that's how it seems to me ... we have nothing as far as activities or opportunities for older people on this estate ... we're very much a forgotten area, what you might call the poor relation in comparison to other areas in the ward (Murray & Crummett, 2018, p. 137).

However, this negative outsider social representation was contrasted with an assertion that the community had many positive features. As one woman recalled:

> They came here with one of these tick-box sheets, and when he'd finished, I said, 'Well, what's the verdict?' And do you know what he said, he said I was deprived. Have you ever heard such rubbish, all of this [indicating her garden] and he said I was deprived (p. 136).

This neighbourhood was their home, and while others might think poorly of it, they recognized the positive features, no matter how limited. Even the negative features of the neighbourhood were recast as evidence of the resilience of the residents.

The community arts project was a means of promoting opportunities for enhanced social engagement. Over a period of several months, the community arts activists worked with a group of older residents in developing a series of art projects. The resultant artworks were displayed to the public in a local exhibition and reported in the local press. The participants not only enjoyed the activities but also began to challenge the negative social representation of their community and of ageing held by both outsiders and the residents themselves. Through media publicity, they began to engage with local officials and demand increased resources.

A related project specifically focused on the potential of community drama. The *Ages and Stages project* 2015 worked with residents of a northern city who had been involved with an innovative local theatre company established in the 1960s. The original aim of that theatre company led by Peter Cheeseman was to challenge the negative social representation of the city. It adopted a form of 'verbatim theatre', in which the scripts for plays were developed from the words of local people (Paget, 1987). Initially, a small group of actors talked with local residents about issues that were impacting their community, such as the closure of a local factory or the run-down of a public service. The actors recorded the interviews and afterwards used these recordings in workshops to develop a dramatic script that conveyed the nature of the local issue. This drama was then performed to local audiences. Sometimes, the performances included an opportunity for audience members to actively participate and express their views. Overall, the aim was for the audience members to become more aware of the underlying issues and even to articulate some form of remedial action. It was a form of conscientization, as promoted in the theatre of the oppressed developed by Boal (1931–2009), the Brazilian theatre activist (Boal, 1979).

The *Ages and Stages project,* led by Mim Bernard (Bernard et al., 2015, 2018), had three acts: first, exploring the original transcripts of the plays performed; second, talking with people who had been involved in the theatre and third, developing a performance about the whole research process. The first stage looked at some of the original scripts to explore how ageing was represented. This initial review of scripts was followed by interviews with some older members of the audience, volunteers at the theatre and a sample of the actors. All of these emphasized the importance of the participatory nature of the theatre in raising their awareness and respect for the local community. Those who had participated in the theatre emphasized that it challenged the dominant negative social representation of ageing and the sense of loss many experienced. Some of the volunteers referred to the renewed sense of purpose that participation in the theatre provided.

Another finding was that, due to exclusion from various activities, everyday life no longer offered a challenge to the older person. Through participation in the theatre the participants felt that they were challenged. As one said:

> I think as you get older, you don't have a manageable challenge ... you're not developing yourself anymore, and I think that's one of the things the

theatre does, not just for young people but for us, It's still developing us, and that's what's so great (p. 100).

This led to the final part of the research, which was the development and production of a dramatic performance. The script was drawn from both the original interviews and workshops with a group of older people/ performers and a group of young people/performers. Thus, the project moved from a consideration of the negative social representation of ageing to the involvement of people in the development of a dramatic performance about ageing that challenged ageist stereotypes.

8.4 Increasing Impact

While community activity focuses on challenging negative social representations in specific communities, minority action can also extend to larger communities in more dispersed locations. This can involve exploring how to widen the impact of minority groups. In a sense, this approach adopts the proverb, 'From little acorns, mighty oaks grow'.

8.4.1 Social Marketing

The converse of the bottom-up community action approach is a more top-down but collaborative approach, which is designed by people in positions of power to change the behaviour of a minority group while taking into consideration its social representations. This social marketing approach was developed by Lauri (2015), based on Kotler and Roberto's (1989) argument that social change depends on understanding the target audience's social environment. Thus, the starting point of any social marketing campaign is researching the social representations held by the target group.

Lauri (2015) reported a study concerned with promoting organ donation in Malta. The study began by conducting focus groups with residents about organ donation. She identified three primary social representations of the body: 'Body belongs to God', 'I own my body' and 'I am my body'. Messages were then developed based on these three representations. Those who believed their body belonged to God were advised that organ donation is an altruistic act supported by church teachings. Those who believed they owned their body were encouraged to let their family know of their wishes and to carry a donor card. The third group, who believed they were their body, were messaged that organ donation gives a new life to recipients.

The campaign that followed was primarily conducted through discussion groups with various groups of residents. These discussion groups identified the primacy of specific representations of organ donation and then tailored their campaign message accordingly. Subsequent research found changes in participants' perceptions of organ donation, and there was also an increase in organ donation, although this could be attributed to a range of factors. Overall, the emphasis was on the need to understand the different social representations.

8.4.2 Media Action

An important factor in the power of minorities is their access to the media. It is through the media that the minority group can promote their message. Marková and Wilkie (1987) explored how a minority group was able to transform a negative view of a particular health-related practice. Initially, when HIV/AIDS was detected in the 1980s, the popular reaction was that it was just retribution for the male homosexual/gay community for engaging in unnatural sexual practices. The gay community reacted strongly and campaigned against this viewpoint. Although they were a minority group, members of this community were often well-educated and articulate men from the arts and media community. They were able to project a counter message that it was not due to their adoption of unnatural sexual practices but the broader acceptance of unsafe sexual practices. Over time, the message to engage in safer sexual practices rather than abstinence was adopted by the health authorities and became more accepted by the general public.

Marková and Wilkie also emphasized the power of the press in subverting the dominant traditional negative moral message. It was often the gay community who were able to articulate their viewpoint through their consistent engagement with the press. This illustrates how a minority group can begin to transform the dominant view of a particular health-related practice. They achieved this through a behavioural style that emphasized consistency, confident and articulate campaigning, an unbiased standpoint by actively obtaining support from the scientific community, and resistance to attempts to denigrate their stance. Those who were expressing this minority viewpoint were not renegades who had been rejected by society but highly regarded individuals who had access to the media, the scientific community, as well as the arts world. Marková and Wilkie (1987) concluded that the impact of this minority group demonstrated that 'social representations are formed, maintained and changed through an interaction of the conservative point of view of society with new ideas of individuals and minorities, disturbing those these may be' (p. 406).

Another study explored the role of the media in subverting dominant negative representations of mental illness (Buchanan & Murray, 2012). People with mental health issues are often excluded from social opportunities. This study organized a community education project with a group of mental health service users (MHSUs) in a city in the English Midlands. It proceeded in three stages. In the first stage, a group of MHSUs participated in a series of group discussions about their social experiences of mental illness. Analysis of the group discussion interview transcripts revealed three primary topics. The first was the hidden nature of mental illness, which, once uncovered, led to changes in how they were treated by others. It was accepted that the dominant social representation of mental illness was very negative. An additional problem was the internalization of this negative representation. As one MHSU said: 'I think there's another kettle when we talk about stigma from society, but also self stigma ... there is such a strong stigma in society we then apply this to ourselves' (p. 38). The second topic was the exclusion from social opportunities and social relationships. As one participant said: 'You do lose friends [leading to] social isolation'. It was felt that the media played a dominant role in perpetuating this negative representation. Another MHSU said: 'The way the media misinterprets everything, it's sort of violence. You know, almost criminal behaviour'. The third topic was the negative representations of mental illness in the media.

In the second stage of the study, a small video project challenging this representation was designed with the former MHSUs. The film critiqued the negative representation in newspapers and television, as well as in everyday social interactions. In the third stage, this film was shown to an audience of local people. The MHSUs were enthused by the project and felt that they had begun to challenge the negative representation not only among others but also among fellow MHSUs. As suggested by Howarth (2006), through coming together in dialogue and debate, the MHSUs in this study began to consider themselves as agents and not as objects. Alone, they felt isolated and powerless, but through working together in developing the video, they grew in confidence. A final example of the role of media action in challenging dominant social representations is the work of Kate Wiskell (2023) which was discussed in Chapter 6. She and her colleagues collected narrative accounts from young people which were subsequently developed into videos for use in media campaigns.

8.5 Changing Times

Throughout history, people have searched to understand their world. This search is the foundation not just of science but of everyday life. This book began by considering the ancient search for shared ideas and how these changed over time and place. It finished by reflecting on the stability and change within these shared ideas. The important point, which was emphasized by Vico, is that people are not pawns in the sway of ideas but rather that we can play a vital part in both constructing them and challenging them.

Social representation theory developed during a time of crisis in Western society. It was, in many ways, a challenge to the dismissal of the everyday lives and thoughts of ordinary people. The aim was *to rehabilitate common thinking and common knowledge* (Moscovici & Marková, 1998, p. 376). Over the past 60 years and more since its development, it has spawned much research. It is an approach that has a heritage but is also in constant development. It provides a framework for making sense of our world today, but it is being refined as it engages with new ideas. One of the strengths of this approach is that, although it is basically social psychological, it connects with other social theories and provides a framework for an interdisciplinary understanding of the world.

In the field of health, biomedical ideas have attained dominance. As Herzlich and Pierret (1987) remarked: 'The discourse of medicine about illness is so loud that it tends to drown out all the others' (p. xi). However, other ideas continue to clash. The development of social representations of health and illness is linked to the changing circumstances of young people. Children are born into a world where scientific medicine has gained prominence as the most important way to understand health and illness. Through everyday social interaction, they gain a broader understanding of health, themselves and their society. As they develop, they become more aware of particular health problems. Once again, in interaction with others, the media and the broader cultural sphere, they gain an understanding of these and react to their experience of these health problems accordingly. Ancient ideas about health and illness are not forgotten but continue to influence our everyday interactions.

Social representations of health and illness are not fixed but change over time and can also be influenced by different forces and events in society. Society is constantly in flux. At the outset, we referred to Moscovici's (1993) concern about the character of modern society, expressed in his book *The Invention of Society*. He remarked that 'modernity has ravaged the European continent through its industries, destroying the bonds that held us together' (p. 69). Taylor (1991) has extended this discussion by itemizing what he termed the three malaises of modernity. The first is the increasing rise of individualism (Santos et al., 2017). This malaise results in individual achievement being considered paramount over the broader social and environmental impact. The second malaise is the rise of instrumental reason, by which he meant that success is measured in terms of short-term cost-benefits. This instrumental reason has promoted the search for technological solutions to all human problems. It has pervaded medical care, where biomedical solutions to all health problems are foremost. The third malaise is the spread of the former two malaises to political life and the consequences for society. Karl Marx has argued in *The Communist Manifesto* (1845) that one of the results of capitalist development is that 'all that is solid melts into air'. Taylor continues: 'The claim is that the solid, lasting, often expressive objects that served us in the past are being set aside for the quick, shoddy, replaceable commodities with which we surround ourselves' (pp. 6–7). Admittedly, there have been many great developments within modernity, such as increased life expectancy. Taylor concludes by remarking, 'As Pascal said about human beings, modernity is characterized by *grandeur* as well as by *misère*' (p. 121). However, with the growth of artificial intelligence the ground is shifting rapidly and the future is more uncertain.

This book was designed to provide an orientation to these changing times. It was not intended to impose a framework but rather to consider ways of making sense of these changes. Moscovici (1993) concluded his book *The Invention of Society* by referring to the verse of the French poet Paul Valéry: 'The wind is rising ... we must try to live' ['*Le vent se lève ... il faut tenter de vivre*']. Earlier in that poem, Valéry writes: 'No, no! Arise! The future years unfold. |Shatter, O body, meditation's mould!" *['Non, non! ... Debout! Dans l'ère successive!| Brisez, mon corps, cette forme pensive!'*] How we understand health and illness will continue to change as society changes. The challenge remains for social psychology to grasp these social and health changes and contribute to a better life for all.

References

Asch, S. E. (1951). Effects of group pressure upon the modification and distortion of judgment. In H. Guetzkow (Ed.), *Groups, Leadership and Men* (pp. 177–190). Carnegie Press.

Balshem, M. (1990). Cancer, control and causality: Talking about cancer in a working class community. *American Ethnologist, 18*(1), 152–172.

Becker, J. C., Hartwich, L., & Haslam, S. A. (2021). Neoliberalism can reduce well-being by promoting a sense of social disconnection, competition, and loneliness. *British Journal of Social Psychology, 60*(3), 947–965.

Bernard, M., Amigoni, D., Basten, R., Munro, L., Murray, M., Reynolds, J., Rezzano, J., & Rickett, M. (2018). The place of theatre in representations of ageing. In A. Walker (Ed.), *The New Dynamics of Ageing* (Vol. 2, pp. 189–215). Policy Press.

Bernard, M., Rickett, M., Amigoni, D., Munro, L., Murray, M., & Rezzano, J. (2015). Ages and stages: The place of theatre in the lives of older people. *Ageing and Society, 35*, 1119–1145.

Billington, J. (2016). *Is literature healthy?* Oxford University Press.

Boal, A. (1979). *Theatre of the oppressed.* London: Pluto.

Bond, H. K. (2000). *The first biography of Jesus: Genre and meaning in Mark's Gospel.* William Eerdmans.

Buchanan, A., & Murray, M. (2012). Using participatory video to challenge the stigma of mental illness: A case study. *International Journal of Mental Health Promotion, 14*, 35–43.

Campbell, C. (2014). Community mobilization in the twenty-first century: Updating our theory of social change? *Journal of Health Psychology, 19*(1), 46–59.

Campbell, C., & Cornish, F. (2014). Reimagining community health psychology: Maps, journeys and new terrains. *Journal of Health Psychology, 19*(1), 3–15.

Campbell, C., & Murray, M. (2004). Community health psychology: Promoting analysis and action for social change. *Journal of Health Psychology, 9*(2), 187–195.

Casey, B., & Murray, M. (2022). Arts-based approaches in social science research. In U. Flick (Ed.), *SAGE handbook of qualitative research design* (pp. 517–534). Sage.

Castro, P., & Mouro, C. (2011). Psycho-social processes in dealing with legal innovation in the community: Insights from biodiversity conservation. *American Journal of Community Psychology, 47*, 362–373.

Doise, W. (1986). *Levels of explanation in social psychology.* Cambridge University Press.

Fallon, D. (2016). Putting the language of pearse in context: Blood sacrifice and 1916. *Irish Independent*, 10.
FISH Safety Foundation. (2022). *Triggering death*. http://www.fishsafety.org
Freire, P. (1994). *The pedagogy of hope: Reliving the pedagogy of the oppressed*. Continuum.
Freire, P. ([1968] 1997). *The pedagogy of the oppressed*. Continuum.
Guareschi, P. A., & Jovchelovitch, S. (2004). Participation, health and the development of community resources in Southern Brazil. *Journal of Health Psychology, 9*(2), 311–322.
Hearn, J., de Boise, S., & Goedecke, K. (2023). Men and masculinities: Structures, practices, and identities. In E. L. Zurbriggen & R. Capdevila (Eds.), *The palgrave handbook of power, gender, and psychology*. Palgrave Macmillan.
Herzlich, C., & Pierret, J. (1987). *Illness and self in society*. Johns Hopkins University Press.
Himmelweit, H. (1990). Societal psychology: Implications and scope. In H. T. Himmelweit & G. Gaskell (Eds.), *Societal psychology* (pp. 17–45). Sage.
Howarth, C. (2006). A social representation is not a quiet thing: Exploring the critical potential of social representations theory. *British Journal of Social Psychology, 45*(1), 65–86.
Howarth, C., Campbell, C., Cornish, F., et al. (2013). Insights from societal psychology: The contextual politics of change. *Journal of Social and Political Psychology, 1*(1), 364–384.
Howarth, C., Foster, J., & Dorrer, N. (2004). Exploring the potential of the theory of social representations in community-based health research—And vice-versa? *Journal of Health Psychology, 9*(2), 229–243.
Hubble, N., & Tew, P. (2013). *Ageing, narrative and identity: New qualitative social research*. Palgrave.
Jodelet, D. (2012). Interconnections between social representations and intervention. In A. de Rosa (Ed.), *Social Representations in the 'Social Arena'* (pp. 77–88). Routledge.
Joffe, H., & Bettega, N. (2004). Social representation of AIDS among Zambian adolescents. *Journal of Health Psychology, 8*(5), 616–631.
Joffe, H., & Haarhoff, G. (2002). Representations of far-flung illnesses: The case of Ebola in Britain. *Social Science and Medicine, 54*(6), 955–969.
Jovchelovitch, S. (2007). *Knowledge in context: Representations, community and culture*. Routledge.
Jovchelovitch, S. (2019). The power of the idea: The legacy of Moscovici. In N. Kalampalikis, D. Jodelet, M. Wieviorka, D. Moscovici, & P. Moscovici (Eds.), *Serge Moscovici: Un Regard Sur Les Mondes Communs* (pp. 165–173). Éditions de la Maison des sciences de l'homme.

Jovchelovitch, S., & Gervais, M. C. (1999). Social representations of health and illness: The case of the Chinese community in England. *Journal of Community and Applied Social Psychology, 9*, 247–260.

Kmietovicz, Z. (2002). R.E.S.P.E.C.T.—Why doctors are still getting enough of it. *BMJ, 324*(7328), 11.

Kotler, P., & Roberto, E. (1989). *Social marketing: Strategies for changing public behaviour*. Free Press.

Krause, M. (2003). The transformation of social representations of chronic disease in a self-help group. *Journal of Health Psychology, 8*(5), 599–615.

Lauri, M. A. (2015). Social change, social marketing and social representations. In G. Sammut, E. Andreouli, G. Gaskell, & J. Valsiner (Eds.), *The Cambridge handbook of social representations* (pp. 397–410). Cambridge University Press.

Marková, I., & Wilkie, P. (1987). Representations, concepts and social change: The phenomenon of AIDS. *Journal for the Theory of Social Behaviour, 17*(4), 389–409.

Marx, K. ([1852] 1968). *The eighteenth Brumaire of Louis Bonaparte*. Progress.

Menezes, D., Woolrych, R., Sixsmith, J., Smith, H., Fisher, J., Garcia-Ferrari, S., Makita, M., Lawthorn, R., Henderson, J., & Murray, M. (2023). "You really do become invisible": Examining older adults' right to the city in the United Kingdom. *Ageing and Society, 43*(10), 2477–2496.

Moscovici, S. (1979). *Psychologie des minorités actives*. Presses Universitaires de France.

Moscovici, S. (1984). The phenomenon of social representations. In R. M. Farr & S. Moscovici (Eds.), *Social representations* (pp. 3–70). Cambridge University Press.

Moscovici, S. (1993). *The invention of society*. Polity.

Moscovici, S. (2000). *Social representations: Explorations in social psychology* (G. Duveen, Ed.). Polity.

Moscovici, S. ([1976] 2008). Psychoanalysis: Its image and its public. In *English translation of la psychoanalyse, son image et son image, 1976*. Polity Press.

Moscovici, S., & Marková, I. (1998). Presenting social representations: A conversation. *Culture and Psychology, 4*(3), 371–410.

Moscovici, S., & Marková, I. (2000). Ideas and their development: A dialogue between Serge Moscovici and Ivana Marková. In S. Moscovici, & G. Duveen (Eds.), *Social representations: Explorations in social psychology* (pp. 208–223). Polity Press.

Murray, M. (2012). Critical health psychology and the scholar-activist tradition. In C. Horrocks & S. E. Johnson (Eds.), *Advances in health psychology: Critical approaches* (pp. 29–43). Palgrave.

Murray, M. (2020). Hidden from view: Some written accounts of community activism. In C. Squire (Ed.), *Stories changing lives. Narratives and paths toward social change* (pp. 75–98). Oxford University Press.

Murray, M., & Campbell, C. (2003). Living in a material world: Reflections on some assumptions of health psychology. *Journal of Health Psychology*, *8*(2), 231–236.

Murray, M., & Crummett, A. (2010). 'I don't think they knew we could do these sorts of things': Social representations of community and participation in community arts by older people. *Journal of Health Psychology*, *15*, 777–785.

Murray, M., & Crummett, A. (2018). Combatting social exclusion through community arts. In A. Walker (ed.), *The new dynamics of ageing* (pp. 129–146). Policy Press.

Murray, M., & Dolomount, M. (1994). *A constant danger: Accidents among fishermen*. Division of Community Health, Memorial University.

Murray, M., Nelson, G., Poland, B., Maticka-Tyndale, E., & Ferris, L. (2004). Assumptions and values in community health psychology. *Journal of Health Psychology*, *9*(2), 315–326.

Murray, M., & Tilley, N. (2006). Using community arts to promote awareness of safety in fishing communities: An action research study. *Safety Science*, *44*, 797–808.

Murray, M., & Ziegler, F. (2015). The narrative psychology of community health workers. *Journal of Health Psychology*, *20*, 338–349.

Negura, L., Plante, N., & Lévesque, M. (2020). The role of social representations in the construction of power relations. *Journal for the Theory of Social Behaviour*, *50*(1), 29–41.

Nemeth, C. B. (1995). Dissent as driving cognition, attitudes, and judgements. *Social Cognition*, *13*(3), 273–291.

Nolas, S.-M. (2014). Towards a new theory of practice for community health psychology. *Journal of Health Psychology*, *19*(1), 126–136.

Paget, D. (1987). 'Verbatim theatre': Oral history and documentary techniques. *New Theatre Quarterly*, *3*(12), 317–336.

Power, S. (2018). Economic inequality and the rise of civic discontent: Deprivation and remembering in an Irish case study. In B. Wagoner, F. N. Moghaddam, & J. Valsiner (Eds.), *The psychology of radical social change: From rage to revolution* (pp. 29–53). Cambridge University Press.

Putnam, R. D. (2000). *Bowling alone: The collapse and revival of American community*. Simon & Schuster.

Reed, J.-P. (2017). The Bible, religious storytelling and revolution: The case of Solentiname, Nicaragua. *Critical Research in Religion*, *5*(3), 227–250.

Santos, H. C., Varnum, M. E. W., & Grossmann, I. (2017). Global increases in individualism. *Psychological Science*, *28*(9), 1228–1239.

Selbin, E. (2010). *Revolution, rebellion, resistance: The power of story*. Zed Books.

Seymour, R., & Murray, M. (2016). When I am old I shall wear purple: A qualitative study of the effect of group poetry sessions on the well-being of older adults. *Working With Older People, 20*(4), 195–198.
Taylor, C. (1991). *The ethics of authenticity*. Harvard University Press.
Walker, A. (Ed.). (2014). *The new science of ageing*. Policy.
Watson, M. (1999). *Lives of their own: Rhetorical dimensions in autobiographies of women activists*. University of South Carolina Press.
Webster, M., & Buglass, G. (2005). *Finding voices, making choices: Creativity for social change*. Educational Heretics Press.

Index

M. Murray, *Social Representations, Health and Illness*,
https://doi.org/10.1007/978-3-031-98494-5

W

FSC
www.fsc.org
MIX
Papier | Fördert
gute Waldnutzung
FSC® C083411

Kolibri 360 GmbH
Ferdinand-Jühlke-Straße 7
99095 Erfurt, Deutschland
produktsicherheit@kolibri360.de